THE
CONTROVERSIAL
CLIMACTERIC

THE CONTROVERSIAL CLIMACTERIC

The workshop moderators' reports
presented at the
Third International Congress on the Menopause,
held in Ostend, Belgium, in June 1981,
under the auspices of the
International Menopause Society.

Edited by
**P. A. van Keep, W. H. Utian
and A. Vermeulen**
The editors were assisted by Pamela Freebody

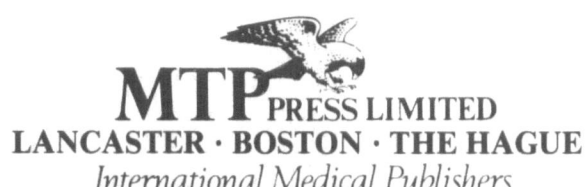
MTP PRESS LIMITED
LANCASTER · BOSTON · THE HAGUE
International Medical Publishers

Published in the UK and Europe by
MTP Press Limited
Falcon House
Lancaster, England

British Library Cataloguing in Publication Data

International Congress on the Menopause (*3rd: 1981: Ostend*)
  The controversial climacteric.
  1. Climacteric – Congresses
  I. Title   II. Keep, P.A. van   III. Utian, W.H.   IV. Vermeulen, A.
  V. International Menopause Society
  612'.665   RC884
  ISBN-13: 978-94-011-7255-4   e-ISBN-13: 978-94-011-7253-0
  DOI: 10.1007/978-94-011-7253-0

Published in the USA by
MTP Press
A division of Kluwer Boston Inc
190 Old Derby Street
Hingham, MA 02043, USA

Library of Congress Cataloging in Publication Data

International Congress on the Menopause (3rd: 1981 : Ostend, Belgium)
  The controversial climacteric.

  Includes index.
  1. Menopause—Congresses.   I. Keep, Pieter A. van.   II. Utian, Wulf H., 1939–
III. Vermeulen, A. (Alex), 1927–   IV. International Menopause Society.
V. Title. [DNLM: 1. Climacteric—Congresses. W3 IN667 3rd 1981s/WP 580 I61 1981c
RG186.I57   1981   618.1'75   82-256
ISBN-13: 978-94-011-7255-4   AACR2

Typeset by Swiftpages Ltd., Liverpool

Contents

Principal contributors

T. Abe
Tohoku University School of Medicine,
Department of Obstetrics and
  Gynaecology,
1-1 Seiryo-machi,
Sendai 980, Japan

P. Aschheim
INSERM, U. 118,
Unité de Recherches Gérontologiques,
29 rue Wilhem,
75016 Paris, France

S. Ballinger
University of Sydney,
Department of Behavioural Sciences,
Sydney, NSW 2006, Australia

F. Bayard
INSERM, U. 168,
Laboratoire d'Endocrinologie
  Expérimentale,
C.H.U. Rangueil,
Chemin du Vallon,
31054 Toulouse Cedex, France

E. W. Bergink
Organon International B. V.,
Scientific Development Group,
P.O. Box 20,
5340 BH Oss, The Netherlands

O. L. M. Bijvoet
Academisch Ziekenhuis Leiden,
Afdeling Klinische Endocrinologie,
Rijnsburgerweg 10,
2333 AA Leiden, The Netherlands

J. Botella Llusiá
Universidad Complutense de Madrid,
Departamento de Obstetricia y
  Ginecologia,
Planta 5° Norte,
Ciudad Universitaria,
Madrid 3, Spain

F. Bottiglioni
Università di Bologna,
Istituto di Patologia Ostetrica e
  Ginecologica,
Policlinico S. Orsola,
Via Massarenti 13,
40138 Bologna, Italy

J. P. Bourguignon
Université de Liège,
Clinique Pédiatrique,
66 boulevard de la Constitution,
4020 Liège, Belgium

P. F. Brenner
University of Southern California School
  of Medicine,
Department of Obstetrics and
  Gynecology,
Women's Hospital,
1240 North Mission Road,
Los Angeles, CA 90033, USA

R. D. Bulbrook
Imperial Cancer Research Fund
  Laboratories,
Department of Clinical Endocrinology,
P.O. Box 123,
Lincoln's Inn Fields,
London WC2A 3PX, UK

P. M. H. G. Buytaert
Universitaire Instelling Antwerpen,
Afdeling Obstetrie en Gynaecologie,
2000 Antwerpen, Belgium

S. Campbell
King's College Hospital Medical School,
Department of Obstetrics and
  Gynaecology,
Denmark Hill,
London SE5 8RX, UK

E. Cohen
Hasharon Hospital,
7 Keren-Kayamet-Le-Israel Street,
Petah-Tiqva, Israel

A. Collin
Leicester Polytechnic,
P.O. Box 143,
Leicester LE1 9BH, UK

D. Cramer
Boston Hospital for Women,
Division of the Brigham and Women's
  Hospital and Harvard Medical School,
75 Francis Street,
Boston, MA 02115, USA

M. G. Crane
Loma Linda University,
Loma Linda, CA 92350, USA

N. Crona
University of Göteborg,
Department of Obstetrics and
  Gynecology,
Sahlgrenska Sjukhuset,
413 45 Göteborg, Sweden

D. A. Davey
University of Cape Town Medical School,
Department of Obstetrics and
  Gynaecology,
Observatory,
7925 Cape, South Africa

A. Demoulin
Université de Liège,
Clinique Gynécologique et Obstétricale,
81 boulevard de la Constitution,
4020 Liège, Belgium

L. Dennerstein
University of Melbourne,
Department of Psychiatry,
Clinical Sciences Building,
c/o P.O. Royal Melbourne Hospitals,
Melbourne, Victoria 3050, Australia

J. G. van Dijk
Academisch Ziekenhuis Leiden,
Vrouwenkliniek,
Gebouw 35 A,
Rijnsburgerweg 10,
2333 AA Leiden, The Netherlands

C. D. van der Does
Diaconessenhuis,
Afdeling Gynaecologie,
Houtlaan 55,
2334 CK Leiden, The Netherlands

N. Dombrowicz
Pepermanstraat 9,
4100 Seraing, Belgium

J. Donnez
Université Catholique de Louvain,
Cliniques Universitaires Saint-Luc,
Département de Gynécologie-
  Obstétrique,
10 avenue Hippocrate,
1200 Bruxelles, Belgium

B. Ehret
Kliniken am Burggraben,
Abteilung Gynäkologie,
Alte Vlothoerstrasse 65,
4902 Bad Salzuflen, West Germany

F. Elkik
Hôpital Broussais,
Clinique Médicale Propédeutique,
96 rue Didot,
75674 Paris Cedex 14, France

L. Fåhraeus
University Hospital,
Department of Obstetrics and
  Gynaecology,
581 85 Linköping, Sweden

E. Fairhurst
University of Manchester,
Department of Geriatric Medicine,
University Hospital of South Manchester,
Nell Lane,
Manchester M20 8LR, UK

M. Featherstone
Teesside Polytechnic,
Department of Social Studies,
Middlesbrough, Cleveland B1 3BA, UK

M. Flint
Montclair State College,
Department of Anthropology,
Upper Montclair, NJ 07043, USA

G. Forti
Università di Firenze,
Scoula di Specializzazione in
  Endocrinologia,
Via Morgagni 85,
50134 Firenze, Italy

P. Franchimont
Université de Liège,
Institut de Médecine,
Laboratoire de Radioimmunologie,
Tour de Pathologie,
C.H.U. – Bâtiment B23,
Sart Tilman par Liège 1, Belgium

R. D. Gambrell
Medical College of Georgia,
Department of Obstetrics and
  Gynecology,
Augusta, GA 30912, USA

U. J. Gaspard
Université de Liège,
Faculté de Médecine,
Clinique Gynécologique et Obstétricale,
81 boulevard de la Constitution,
4020 Liège, Belgium

A. R. Genazzani
Università degli Studi di Siena,
Cattedra di Patologia Ostetrica e
  Ginecologica,
Via Pietro Mascagni 4,
53100 Siena, Italy

C. Gold
University of Toronto,
Toronto General Hospital,
1849 Yonge Street, Suite 307,
Toronto, Canada M4S 1Y2

L. Goldie
The Royal Marsden Hospital (London
  and Surrey),
Fulham Road,
London SW3 6JJ, UK

R. B. Greenblatt
Medical College of Georgia
School of Medicine,
Department of Endocrinology,
Augusta, GA 30901, USA

M. van Haaften
Academisch Ziekenhuis Utrecht,
Afdeling Endocrinologie,
Catharijnesingel 101,
3500 CG Utrecht, The Netherlands

J. Hailes
Royal Women's Hospital,
Menopause Clinic,
Melbourne, Victoria, Australia

E. V. van Hall
Academisch Ziekenhuis Leiden,
Rijnsburgerweg 10,
2333 AA Leiden, The Netherlands

A. A. Haspels
Academisch Ziekenhuis Utrecht,
Universiteitskliniek voor Obstetrie en
  Gynaecologie,
Catharijnesingel 101,
3500 CG Utrecht, The Netherlands

R. P. Heaney
Creighton University,
Department of Medicine,
2500 California Street,
Omaha, NE 68178, USA

J. H. C. L. Hendriks
Katholieke Universiteit,
Sint Radboudziekenhuis,
Instituut voor Röntgendiagnostiek,
Geert Groteplein Zuid 18,
6500 HB Nijmegen, The Netherlands

M. Hepworth
University of Aberdeen,
Department of Sociology,
Edward Wright Building,
Dunbar Street,
Old Aberdeen AB9 2TY, UK

E. Hirvonen
University Central Hospital,
Department of Obstetrics and
  Gynaecology,
00290 Helsinki 29, Finland

F. A. Holstein
Universität Hamburg,
Universitäts-Krankenhaus Eppendorf,
Abteilung Mikroskopische Anatomie,
Martinistrasse 52,
2000 Hamburg 20, West Germany

A. Holte
University of Oslo,
Institute of Psychology,
P.B. 1094, Blindern,
Oslo 3, Norway

H. S. Jacobs
St. Mary's Hospital Medical School,
Paddington,
London W2 1PG, UK

V. H. T. James
St. Mary's Hospital Medical School,
Department of Chemical Pathology,
Paddington,
London W2 1PG, UK

H. L. Judd
University of California,
Los Angeles School of Medicine,
Department of Obstetrics and
  Gynecology,
Center for the Health Sciences,
Los Angeles, CA 90024, USA

P. A. van Keep
International Health Foundation,
8 avenue Don Bosco,
1150 Bruxelles, Belgium

R. J. B. King
Imperial Cancer Research Fund
  Laboratories,
Department of Hormone Biochemistry,
P.O. Box 123,
Lincoln's Inn Fields,
London WC2A 3PX, UK

G. Langer
Psychiatrische Universitätsklinik,
14 Lazarettgasse,
1097 Wien, Austria

U. Larsson-Cohn
University Hospital,
Department of Obstetrics and
  Gynaecology,
581 85 Linköping, Sweden

C. Lauritzen
Universität Ulm,
Frauenklinik,
Prittwitzstrasse 43,
7900 Ulm/Donau, West Germany

R. F. Lax
1185 Park Avenue,
New York, NY 10028, USA

C. Lecart
Université Catholique de Louvain,
Cliniques Universitaires Saint-Luc,
Département de Gynécologie-
  Obstétrique,
10 avenue Hippocrate,
1200 Bruxelles, Belgium

B. de Lignières
Hôpital Necker,
Service d'Endocrinologie et de
  Gynécologie Médicale,
149 rue de Sèvres,
75730 Paris Cedex 15, France

M. A. Limouzin-Lamothe
Hôpital Bichat,
34 avenue Hoche,
75008 Paris, France

R. Lindsay
Helen Hayes Hospital,
Regional Bone Center,
Route 9W,
West Haverstraw, NY 10993, USA

P. Linkowski
Université de Bruxelles,
Département de Psychiatrie,
Hôpital Erasme,
808 route de Lennik,
1070 Bruxelles, Belgium

J. McQueen
Beckenham Hospital,
379 Croydon Road,
Beckenham, Kent BR3 3QL, UK

B. Maoz
Ben-Gurion University of the Negev,
Soroka Medical Center,
P.O. Box 151,
Beer Sheva 84120, Israel

F. Michiels
Parklaan 55,
2700 Sint Niklaas, Belgium

A. Mikkelsen
University of Oslo,
Institute of Behavioural Sciences in
   Medicine,
P.O. Box 1111, Blindern,
Oslo 3, Norway

G. Milhaud
Hôpital Saint Antoine,
Service de Médecine Nucléaire,
184 rue du Faubourg Saint Antoine,
75571 Paris Cedex 12, France

H. van der Molen
Erasmus Universiteit,
Afdeling Chemische Endocrinologie,
P.O. Box 1738,
3000 DR Rotterdam, The Netherlands

H. Molinski
Universitäts-Frauenklinik Düsseldorf,
Psychosomatische Abteilung,
Moorenstrasse 5,
4000 Düsseldorf, West Germany

B. Moore
Dudley Road Hospital,
Department of Obstetrics and
   Gynaecology,
Dudley Road,
Birmingham B18 7QH, UK

H. Musaph
Academisch Ziekenhuis Utrecht,
Universiteitskliniek voor Obstetrie en
   Gynaecologie,
Catharijnesingel 101,
3500 CG Utrecht, The Netherlands

J. Need
Flinders Medical Centre,
Department of Obstetrics and
   Gynaecology,
Bedford Park, South Australia 5042,
Australia

M. Neves-e-Castro
Organon International B.V.,
Scientific Development Group,
P.O. Box 20,
5340 BH Oss, The Netherlands

B. E. C. Nordin
MRC Mineral Metabolism Unit,
The General Infirmary,
Great George Street,
Leeds LS1 3EX, UK

M. Notelovitz
The Center for Climacteric Studies,
University of Florida,
The Professional Center,
901 NW 8th Avenue, Suite B-1,
Gainesville, FL 32601, USA

J. Ovadia
The Beilinson Medical Center,
Beilinson Hospital,
Petah-Tiqva, Israel

J. R. Pasqualini
C.N.R.S. Steroid Hormone Research
   Unit,
Foundation for Hormone Research,
26 boulevard Brune,
75014 Paris, France

J. Poortman
Academisch Ziekenhuis Utrecht,
Universiteitskliniek voor Inwendige
  Geneeskunde,
Klinische Endocrinologie,
Catharijnesingel 101,
3500 CG Utrecht, The Netherlands

L. Rauramo
University of Turku,
Department of Obstetrics and
  Gynaecology,
Kaskenkatu II B,
20700 Turku 70, Finland

C. Richards
Caerphilly District Miners' Hospital,
St. Martins Road,
Caerphilly CF8 2WW, UK

B. L. Riggs
Mayo Clinic,
Department of Endocrinology and
  Internal Medicine,
Rochester, MN 55901, USA

H. Roberts
Ilkley College,
Wells Road,
Ilkley, West Yorkshire LS29 9RD, UK

G. Samsioe
University of Göteborg,
Department of Obstetrics and
  Gynecology,
Sahlgrenska Sjukhuset,
413 45 Göteborg, Sweden

P. Sarrel
Yale University School of Medicine,
333 Cedar Street,
New Haven, CT 06510, USA

L. Schenkel
Ciba-Geigy AG,
4002 Basel, Switzerland

I. Schiff
Boston Hospital for Women,
Division of the Brigham and Women's
  Hospital and Harvard Medical School,
75 Francis Street,
Boston, MA 02115, USA

A. E. Schindler
Eberhard-Karls-Universität Tübingen,
Universitäts-Frauenklinik,
7400 Tübingen-1, West Germany

H. Schmidt
Klinik für Diagnostik,
Aukammallee 33,
6200 Wiesbaden, West Germany

H. P. G. Schneider
Universitäts-Frauenklinik,
Westring 11,
4400 Münster, West Germany

B. von Schoultz
University of Umeå,
Department of Obstetrics and
  Gynaecology,
901 87 Umeå, Sweden

M. de Senarclens
1 place de la Taconnerie,
1204 Genève, Switzerland

D. M. Serr
The Chaim Sheba Medical Center,
Division of Obstetrics and Gynecology,
Tel-Hashomer, Israel

E. G. C. van Seumeren
Academisch Ziekenhuis Utrecht,
Universiteitskliniek voor Obstetrie en
  Gynaecologie,
Catharijnesingel 101,
3500 CG Utrecht, The Netherlands

N. C. Siddle
King's College Hospital Medical School,
Department of Obstetrics and
  Gynaecology,
Denmark Hill,
London SE5 8RX, UK

R. Sitruk-Ware
Hôpital Necker,
Service d'Endocrinologie et de
  Gynécologie Médicale,
149 rue de Sèvres,
75730 Paris Cedex 15, France

M. Smith
University of Western Australia,
Midlands, West Australia 6009, Australia

J. Stevenson
Royal Postgraduate Medical School,
Hammersmith Hospital,
Ducane Road,
London W12 OHS, UK

J. W. W. Studd
King's College Hospital,
Department of Obstetrics and
   Gynaecology,
Denmark Hill,
London SE5 8RX, UK

D. Sturdee
University Department of Obstetrics and
   Gynaecology,
Birmingham Maternity Hospital,
Birmingham B15 TG, UK

P. F. Tauber
Universitätsklinikum Essen,
Frauenklinik und Poliklinik,
Hufelandstrasse 55,
4300 Essen 1, West Germany

J. H. H. Thijssen
Academisch Ziekenhuis Utrecht,
Universiteitskliniek voor Inwendige
   Geneeskunde,
Klinische Endocrinologie,
Catharijnesingel 101,
3500 CG Utrecht, The Netherlands

A. Treloar
9714 Campana Drive,
Sun City, AZ 85351, USA

L. Tseng
State University of New York at Stony
   Brook,
Department of Obstetrics and
   Gynecology,
Stony Brook, NY 11794, USA

W. H. Utian
The Mount Sinai Hospital of Cleveland,
Department of Obstetrics-Gynecology,
University Circle,
Cleveland, OH 44106, USA

W. H. M. van der Velden
St. Josephziekenhuis,
Afdeling Gynaecologie en Obstetrie,
Aalsterweg 259,
5600 ML Eindhoven, The Netherlands

A. Vermeulen
Rijksuniversiteit Gent,
Akademisch Ziekenhuis,
Dienst voor Inwendige Ziekten,
Afdeling Endocrinologie, Hematologie,
   Stofwisselingszieten,
De Pintelaan 135,
9000 Gent, Belgium

M. P. Vessey
University of Oxford,
Department of Community Medicine and
   General Practice,
8 Keble Road,
Oxford OX1 3QN, UK

J. van der Vies
Organon International B.V.,
Endocrinological R & D Laboratories,
P.O. Box 20,
5340 BH Oss, The Netherlands

A. Vizzotto
International Health Foundation,
Via Fabio Filzi 23,
20124 Milano, Italy

K. D. Voigt
Universität Hamburg,
Universitäts-Krankenhaus Eppendorf,
Abteilung für Klinische Chemie,
Martinistrasse 52,
2000 Hamburg 20, West Germany

H. Wauters
St. Camillus Kliniek,
Lockaertstraat 10,
Antwerpen, Belgium

M. I. Whitehead
King's College Hospital Medical School,
Department of Obstetrics and
   Gynaecology,
Denmark Hill,
London SE5 8RX, UK

M. A. H. M. Wiegerinck
St. Josephziekenhuis,
Afdeling Gynaecologie en Obstetrie,
Aalsterweg 259,
5600 ML Eindhoven, The Netherlands

J. Wilbush
Apt. 36, 11112, 129th Street,
Edmonton, Alberta T5M OY5, Canada

B. Wren
Royal Hospital for Women,
Menopause Clinic,
Paddington, Sydney, NSW 2021,
Australia

L. Zichella
Università di Roma,
IVª Cattedra di Patologia Ostetrica e
   Ginecologica,
Policlinico Umberto 1,
00161 Roma, Italy

Preface

Three International Congresses on the Menopause have been held during the last five years, evidence of the explosive increase in the scientific study of this subject. The first, held in La Grande Motte, near Montpellier, France, in June 1976, was designed to provide a consensus on menopause research (van Keep *et al.*, 1976). The second, held in Jerusalem, was planned to assess the developing research (van Keep *et al.*, 1979).

The objective of the third congress, convened in June 1981 in Ostend, Belgium, under the auspices of the International Menopause Society, was to explore areas of controversy in basic understanding and in the therapeutic advances relating to the climacteric.

The workshop moderators were selected because of their acknowledged leadership in menopause research, and each was invited to arrange a workshop on a specific area of interest or concern. The moderators, whilst being given a free hand as far as the selection of invited speakers was concerned, were asked to allow plenty of time for open discussion. In particular, they were encouraged to stimulate debate about controversial issues.

The only plenary session of the congress was held on the final afternoon of the three-day meeting, when each moderator presented a report on the workshop over which he had presided. It is these reports, sometimes slightly elaborated upon, which are presented here. This book therefore represents a comprehensive summation of current thinking on the subject of the climacteric, as presented by over 100 investigators from 17 countries. It also highlights areas in which further research is felt to be needed in order to settle important issues, or, in some instances, to clarify details. It is hoped that the congress itself and this book will act as a catalyst for further investigations, which can perhaps be evaluated in depth at the next congress in this series, which is planned for the USA in 1984.

To a large extent the success of the Third International Congress on the Menopause was due to the expertise and enthusiasm of the workshop moderators who so ably organized and chaired their workshops. We do indeed thank them for this, and, as editors, we also thank them for providing reports for the plenary session and for this book. We thank too the specially invited speakers for their contributions, the people who presented papers during the free communications sessions, and those whose work was reported in the poster sessions. Thanks are also due, and are hereby extended, to all those involved with the organization of the congress, particularly to those who joined us on the Organizing Committee, Drs E. V. van Hall, A. A. Haspels, C. Lecart, F. Michiels and J. H. H. Thijssen, and on the Programme Committee, Drs S. Campbell, R. B. Greenblatt, H. P. G. Schneider, D. M. Serr, R. Sitruk-Ware and L. Zichella. Finally, but most importantly, we thank the people, all 400 of them, who attended the meeting, and who so enthusiastically joined in the various discussion sessions. We hope that they will agree with us that these published proceedings accurately reflect the atmosphere of the meeting, the information presented, and the points of view expressed.

P. A. VAN KEEP
W. H. UTIAN
A. VERMEULEN

References

van Keep, P. A., Greenblatt, R. B. and Albeaux-Fernet, M. (eds.) (1976). *Consensus on Menopause Research*. (Lancaster: MTP Press)

van Keep, P. A., Serr, D. M. and Greenblatt, R. B. (eds.) (1979). *Female and Male Climacteric*. (Lancaster: MTP Press)

Workshop 1

Gonadal function in the ageing male

Moderator: **K. D. Voigt**

Speakers: **G. Forti** (Italy)
F. A. Holstein (West Germany)
H. van der Molen (The Netherlands)
F. F. G. Rommerts (The Netherlands)
H. Schmidt (West Germany)
M. Serio (Italy)
A. Vermeulen (Belgium)

This workshop, on a subject which is clearly one of growing interest, was both lively and thought-provoking.

The first speaker was *Holstein*, whose lecture on 'Do human male germ cells exhibit changes with ageing?' was illustrated with superb electron microscopic pictures. According to *Holstein*, it is indeed possible to see age-related changes in the histology of seminiferous tubuli. In old men there are large variations in tubular diameter and many diverticula of the seminiferous tubuli. Several types of spermatogonia can be observed which are different from the well-known A-pale, A-dark, A-cloudy, and A-long types. There are sometimes clusters of A-spermatogonia which occlude the lumen of the seminiferous tubule. A-spermatogonia leave the basal compartment of the germinal epithelium without having undergone the first changes of the spermatogenetic process. Meiosis may be disturbed and development and maturation of primary spermato-cytes is sometimes arrested at the prophase; these primary germatocytes often degenerate. Multiple abnormalities of spermatids have also been observed, and early spermatid differentiation may be disturbed, leading to the appearance of giant cells spermatids. In addition the relationship between germ cells and Sertoli cells is sometimes impaired, with the spermatids being released from the germinal epithelium before maturation. These changes indicate that the immunological barrier of the germinal epithelium is impaired, an assumption which is further supported by the appearance of spermatophages which eliminate spermatozoa already in the seminiferous tubule. The above-mentioned changes, concerning the organization of the germinal epithelium, the cytology of germ cells, and the relationship between germ cells and Sertoli cells, are all considered to be morphological changes occurring as part of the general ageing process.

The discussion after *Holstein*'s lecture concentrated on the relationship between germ cells and Sertoli cells, and on the clinical significance of the alterations observed.

Rommerts and *van der Molen* then turned the attention of the audience to the biochemical aspects of testicular function and to its changes with age. Their subject was 'Testis function in the ageing rat testis, *in vivo* and *in vitro*'.

It has recently become possible to grow homogenous cell clones in chemically defined culture media. With these preparations the (direct) cellular response to hormones, and other factors, can be investigated under strictly defined conditions. It is true that isolated cells in culture may differ from cells in the original tissue, and that the results obtained with cultured cells may reflect the *potential* of the cells rather than the true *in vivo* situation, but it may also be that investigations of changes occurring in cells in culture will reveal properties which also play a rôle during the ageing of the cells under normal *in vivo* conditions.

In the experiments reported by *Rommerts* and *van der Molen* Leydig cell suspensions were prepared from collagenase-treated testis tissue obtained from immature and from mature rats, and from a rat Leydig cell tumour. These suspensions, sometimes after purification through Ficoll, were pre-incubated for 1 h at 37 °C in petri dishes containing 2 ml culture medium with 1% fetal calf serum. During the pre-incubation period most of the Leydig cells, but not the germinal cells or the erythrocytes, firmly attached to the plastic surfaces. Production of testosterone and of pregnenolone was measured by direct radioimmunoassay of the steroids present in the culture medium (in the presence of inhibitors of pregnenolone metabolism in the latter case).

It was found that production of testosterone by mature Leydig cells during the third hour after the addition of LH was $41 \pm 6\%$ (5) that during the first hour, whereas production of pregnenolone, measured in separate dishes, was virtually unchanged ($110 \pm 28\%$) (5). These results indicate that Leydig cells remain active with respect to pregnenolone production for several hours, whereas their capacity to produce testosterone quickly diminishes, which may indicate that the pregnenolone-converting enzymes located in the microsomes become less active.

Production of testosterone and of pregnenolone by Leydig cells from mature and from tumour testis tissue could not be stimulated with LH after a pre-incubation period of 24 h without LH, although the cells remained morphologically viable for more than 5 days and showed 3β-hydroxysteroid dehydrogenase activity during that period. Immature Leydig cells, however, could be stimulated with LH to produce pregnenolone, but not testosterone, after 24–48 h in culture. After 5 days in culture these immature Leydig cells were inactive as far as pregnenolone production was concerned, but active with respect to 3β-hydroxysteroid dehydrogenase activity, which was also seen immediately after the isolation of the cells, but not between days 2 and 5 in culture.

When Sertoli cells from immature rats were incubated *in vitro* at 37°C the secretion rate of the androgen-binding protein in culture on day 6 in culture was half that seen on day 1. In contrast, the incorporation of [³H]leucine into the secreted proteins was the same on day 6 as it was on day 1. The production of oestradiol from added testosterone was 30-fold higher on day 6 than on day 1. Changes in synthesis of extracellular and intracellular proteins were also observed during the first few culture days.

The alterations in the steroidogenic activities and synthesis or phosphorylation of proteins in the Leydig cells and in the Sertoli cells could represent an adaptation of the isolated testicular cells to the new (culture) environment. It remains to be seen if similar processes are involved in the ageing of the cells under *in vivo* conditions.

The discussion which followed the presentation of this information from *Rommerts* and *van der Molen* centred on the integrity of Leydig cell suspension, and on the problem of whether or not this is a good model for human testicular function.

Forti and *Serio* then reported on their work in measuring steroid concentrations in human spermatic venous blood. While testosterone is almost exclusively secreted by the testis, other androgens and some oestrogens also come from adrenal secretion and/or from the peripheral conversion of precursors. Therefore the measurement of steroids in the spermatic venous blood, taken during surgical intervention for undescended testis or for hernia repair, seemed to *Forti* and *Serio* to be a more direct approach to the problem of measuring age-related changes in testicular hormone secretion *in vivo*.

Testosterone levels in blood obtained in this way were found to be significantly higher than peripheral levels in prepubertal boys affected by cryptorchidism ($n=49$) or by inguinal hernia ($n=10$). Androstenedione levels in this spermatic venous blood were found to be significantly higher than peripheral levels in boys with undescended testis ($n=18$), but not in boys with inguinal hernia ($n=8$). When the two groups of boys were considered together a significant linear relationship was found both (a) between age and testosterone levels ($r=0.6952$, $n=59$, $p<0.01$), and (b) between age and androstenedione levels ($r=0.6323$, $n=26$, $p<0.01$). These data show (1) that the prepubertal human testis secretes both testosterone and androstenedione, and (2) that this testicular secretion is age-related in the prepubertal period.

Spermatic venous blood levels of testosterone, androstenedione, dehydroepiandrosterone, androstenediol and dihydrotestosterone were also measured in a group of 25 men (age range 20–70 years) undergoing surgery for inguinal hernia repair. Using a weighted regression analysis, a significant negative correlation with age was found for all these steroids (testosterone $r=-0.6759$, $p<0.001$; androstenedione $r=-0.6077$, $p<0.01$; dehydroepiandrosterone $r=-0.4881$, $p<0.05$; androstenediol $r=-0.7637$, $p<0.001$; dihydrotestosterone $r=-0.6971$, $p<0.001$). These results show a reduction of testicular androgen secretion with age.

The increase of oestradiol plasma concentrations found by several authors in ageing males seems to be associated with a decreased metabolic clearance rate and an unchanged blood production rate. Since the testicular and adrenal secretion of aromatizable androgens decreases with age, the unchanged blood production rate of oestradiol could be due to an increase in testicular secretion of oestradiol and/or to an increase in the peripheral aromatization of testosterone. No significant variation of oestradiol spermatic concentrations with age was found in the 25 subjects mentioned above. This suggests that the increase of oestradiol in peripheral plasma in ageing males is due partly to the reduced metabolic clearance rate and partly to an increase in peripheral aromatization of androgens. An increase of testicular secretion of oestradiol seems to be excluded. Moreover, as androgen levels in the spermatic venous blood decrease with age, the absence of a decrease of oestradiol in the spermatic venous blood might be explained by an increased aromatization at the testicular level similar to that observed in the other aromatizing tissues.

4

The discussion after the presentation of these data centred on the differences between the findings in peripheral blood to those in spermatic venous blood, on the rôle of the blood flow, and on its influence on the amount of steroid secreted. The clinical relevance of the decreasing androgen production was also discussed.

Vermeulen then drew attention to a new type of investigation in the study of this subject, namely the determination of endogenous androgen concentration in target organ cells. In view of the clinical evidence of decreased androgenicity and of the decrease in plasma free androgen levels in old age, it seemed worthwhile to determine endogenous androgen levels in androgen target and non-target tissues at various ages in man. Accordingly, the following steroids were measured in post-mortem pubic skin, scrotal skin, thigh skin and striated muscle of 24 males aged between 20 and 82; testosterone, 5α-dihydrotestosterone, and 5α-androstanediol.

Androgen concentrations were found to be highest in scrotal skin, followed by pubic skin, and lowest in thigh skin and striated muscle. Using the equation of 5α-dihydrotestosterone plus 5α-androstanediol over testosterone as a parameter of 5α-reductase activity, this activity was similarly found to be highest in scrotal skin, then in pubic skin, thigh skin and striated muscle, in that order. When the 5α-androstanediol over 5α-dihydrotestosterone equation was taken as a parameter of 3α-reductase activity, the activity was highest in striated muscle, then in thigh skin, pubic skin and scrotal skin.

An age-dependent decrease in androgen concentration was found only in pubic skin. When considering the unexpected absence of a decrease in androgen concentration in scrotal skin, one should remember that the same situation is found in the prostate, an organ with a similar embryological origin as the scrotum. The absence of a decrease in androgen concentration in the other tissues studied might be due to the relatively low concentrations found, to high individual variability, and to the small number of subjects studied.

The discussion which followed the presentation of these data showed that many of those present felt that investigations such as these might well provide a better understanding than blood androgen determinations of the pathological changes which occur with age.

The last paper in this session was presented by *Schmidt*, whose topic was 'Clinical aspects of impaired sexual function and climacteric symptoms in the ageing male'.

Schmidt introduced this subject by remarking that, starting in the 1940s, many authors, principally Americans, have published their observations that ageing men can suffer complaints which are similar to those seen in females around the time of the climacteric. As a result, over the years a whole series of psychological complaints and vegetative disorders has come to be thought by some to occur because of biological or pathological decrease in endocrine testicular function. Herrmann and Beach (1976), it must be said, certainly found characteristics of neuroticism and a high level of psychovegetative complaints in patients with androgen deficiency.

It does seem, however, that whereas in the female a relatively sudden change can occur as the result of oestrogen-deficiency after the menopause, in the male there is a slow and continuous increase in psychovegetative problems with age, and not a sudden change in any one period of life. This was certainly the conclusion drawn by Kies (1974) after conducting a large study involving 10 000 male out-patient subjects suffering from so-called 'climacteric' complaints. In a sub-section of that study, an analysis of configuration frequency of 12 problems in nearly 5000 males aged 45 to 65 revealed only three combinations of problems to be related to a higher frequency than expected in a random distribution; these were (1) sexual disturbances and sweating, (2) sexual disturbances and 'nervousness', and (3) constipation and insomnia. Investigations into a possible association between 'climacteric' symptoms and changes in hormonal testicular function were fruitless. Urinary testosterone glucuronide excretion was not found to be significantly diminished in men with 'climacteric' complaints, and mean plasma testosterone levels in these men were found to be the same as in men of the same age but without complaints. In only a few cases did a short time HCG stimulation test result in somewhat low testosterone levels, but no correlation could be found when basal and stimulated testosterone levels were compared with the results of a large series of psychometric tests.

For some time now androgen treatment has been thought by some to be of value in reducing psychovegetative problems in the ageing male, some physicians regarding it as replacement therapy. Many papers have been published supporting this theory, but, unfortunately, few have been soundly based on controlled trials. It is true, however, that androgens have been shown to exert psychotropic effects in males with normal testicular function; the EEG changes seen are similar to those seen after the administration of anti-depressant drugs, and statistically significant effects have been recorded in motoric and performance tests. Beneficial effects have also been seen in chronic depressive patients after the administration of high doses of the androgen mesterolone.

One controlled double-blind study which has been carried out in order to see whether the psychotropic effects of androgen therapy are useful in combating the psychovegetative problems of ageing men is that of Kaiser *et al.* (1978). This study involved 66 men aged between 45 and 66. The psychovegetative problems most frequently recorded on the symptom list used to select subjects for this study were: diminished productivity and disinclination to work, poor concentration, poor memory, listlessness, weariness, unusual fatigability, and increased irritability. A large number of tests was carried out; there was a questionnaire to measure psychovegetative symptomatology, a test to measure the personality factors extroversion and introversion and neuroticism, a multi-dimensional personality test, an adjective check list to assess emotional and affective states, a test designed to measure concentration and performance, and the Critical Flicker Frequency Test was used to determine stimulatory effects on the central nervous system. The tests were performed before treatment, and repeated after a five-week period of treatment during which the subjects received either 75 mg/day mesterolone (34 subjects) or placebo (32 subjects).

The results of the pre-treatment tests, besides confirming the fact that all subjects were suffering various psychovegetative problems, showed the subjects, taken as a group, to rate below normal in the test designed to assess personality; a low score in this test may be said to describe the following character: someone who is quiet, withdrawn, shy, inhibited, of depressed mood, lacking in self-confidence, and suffering various psychosomatic problems.

After the five-week treatment period a multi-variate co-variance analysis revealed a significant difference ($p < 0.01$) between the two treatment groups in favour of mesterolone in connection with a 'test package' describing personality factors, including masculine self-image, but no significant differences between the two groups in connection with test packages describing psychovegetative symptoms, activity and performance, or mood and feeling. A separate analysis of the tendency to change during treatment showed mesterolone to have a favourable influence in tests designed to assess activity and performance, neuroticism, extroversion, and masculine self-image. No correlation could be found between endocrine function and the pre-treatment scores, or between testosterone levels and the pre- and post-treatment results of the psychometric tests. It is the opinion of the investigators that the changes seen are evidence of a psychotropic effect inherent in the androgen administered.

7

The opinion of *Schmidt* that there is a gradual and continuous increase in psychovegetative problems with ageing, but no male climacteric syndrome as such, was by no means unanimously accepted by the audience. Several discussants stuck firmly to their belief that such a syndrome does exist, and argued strongly for its recognition, both for diagnostic and for therapeutic purposes.

In conclusion, it seems clear from this workshop that our knowledge of the histological and biochemical changes which occur in gonadal function with age is increasing rapidly. New methods of investigation are opening new fields of research, and these will undoubtedly further extend our understanding of the physiological processes involved. It seems, however, that we still have some way to go in translating our knowledge into practical aids for diagnostic and therapeutic purposes.

Bibliography

Deslypere, J. P. and Vermeulen, A. (1981). Ageing and tissue androgens. *J. Clin. Endocrinol. Metab.*, **53**, 430

Hammond, G. L. (1978). Endogenous steroid levels in the human prostate from birth to old age: a comparison of normal and diseased tissues. *J. Endocrinol.*, **78**, 7

Herrmann, W. M. and Beach, R. C. (1976). Psychotropic effects of androgens: A review of clinical observations and new human experimental findings. *Pharmakopsychiat.*, **9**, 205

Kaiser, E., Kies, N., Maass, G., Schmidt, H., Beach, R. C., Bormacher, K., Herrmann, W. M. and Richter, E. (1978). The measurement of the psychotropic effects of an androgen in aging males with psychovegetative symptomatology: A controlled double blind study mesterolone versus placebo. *Prog. Neuro-Psychopharmacol.*, **2**, 505

Kies, N. (1974). Die klimakterische Symptomatologie aus klinisch-psychologischer Sicht. *Med. Welt*, **25**, 228

Workshop 2

The pre-menopause

Moderator: **H. P. G. Schneider** (West Germany)

Speakers: **J. Hendriks** (The Netherlands)
             C. Lauritzen (West Germany)
             M. Notelovitz (USA)
             R. Sitruk-Ware (France)
             A. Treloar (USA)
             M. I. Whitehead (UK)

INTRODUCTION

At the outset of this report on the workshop devoted to the pre-menopause it seems wise to explain exactly what is meant by the term 'pre-menopause'. Simply put, *menopause* denotes the final menstrual bleeding. The time closest to this event is called the *peri-menopause*, before that there is the *pre-menopause*, and after it the *post-menopause*. The pre-menopause does not cover the whole of the woman's life before the menopause, but merely the time (a) from around 40 years of age when a woman can reasonably be said to be approaching the menopause, or (b) when a woman feels the approach of the menopause, by experiencing pre-menopausal irregularities in her menstrual cycle or other 'menopausal' or 'climacteric' symptoms.

In this workshop consideration was given to how best to cope with the clinical management of this period of life, which is a time when rather special care is sometimes needed.

THE MENSTRUAL CYCLE DURING THE PRE-MENOPAUSE

Treloar in his Menstrual and Reproductive Health Research Program in Chapel Hill, North Carolina, has been prospectively assembling inform-ation since 1934 on human menstrual history. His study began with a pilot group of 526 students and now embraces two generations of daughters, enroled at the time of menarche. From this supply of data *Treloar* presented a report on 763 cases in which menstrual records, terminating in menopause, have been very precisely kept. It is clear from these records that complete regularity in menstruation for an extended period of time is a myth. Variation is the rule, and exceptions are of short duration. Women apparently use the term 'regular' as they do '28 days' in order to indicate belief that they are normal in their menstrual charac-teristics. The first few years of menstrual life and the last few are usually years of varied patterns of short and long cycles; they are years of

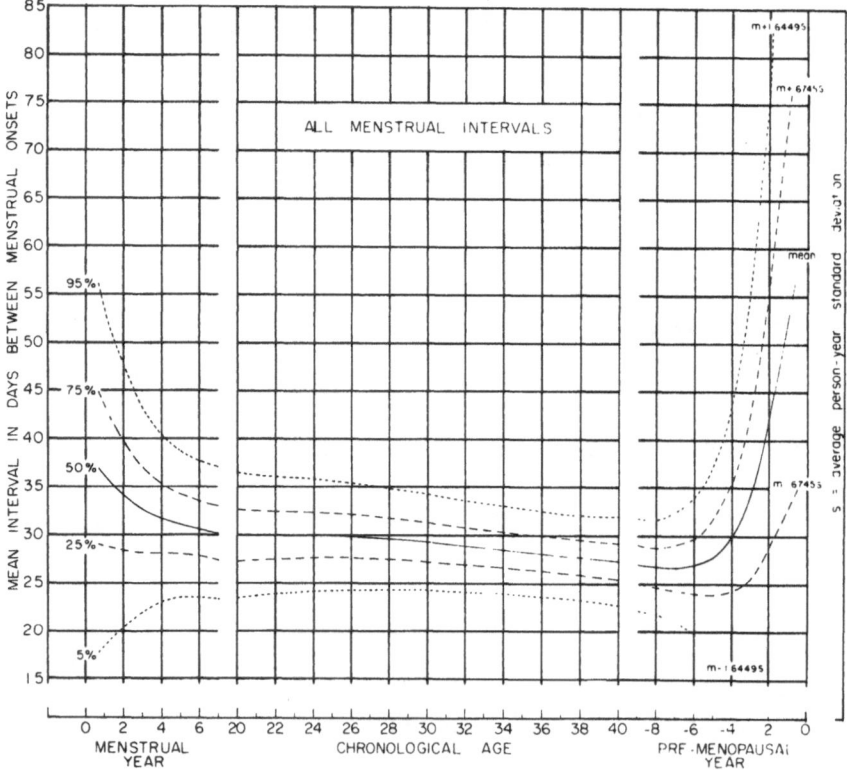

Figure 1 Normal curve contours for the distribution of intervals between onsets of menstrual bleeding in three zones of experience (Treloar *et al.*, 1967)

transition into and out of a relatively more regular pattern in the 'midlife' section (Figure 1).

These periods of transition vary considerably in length, but seem usually to occupy about five to seven years after menarche and six to eight years before menopause. On the contour diagrams of changing frequency distributions with age, these two transition zones are very much like mirror images of one another, with both central trend and variations changing in curvilinear forms.

The midlife section, which may be said to occupy about two decades beginning around the age of twenty, is usually characterized by a general shortening of the intervals between bleedings by two or three days. A persistent increase in variation of longer and shorter than usual flow intervals is the crucial phenomenon characterizing the transition to menopause. The shorter intervals counterbalance the longer ones for a while, the median length of interval does not increase right away, whereas the range of variation in intervals becomes progressive without delay. This latter feature presents an analogy to detection of something going wrong in industrial manufacturing for which statistical methods of quality control have been developed. Adapting these methods to menstrual cycle variations has demonstrated that prevalence of the pre-menopausal period can be detected shortly after its onset. Having determined an individual's entrance into the menopausal transition, a record keeper may then like to ascertain the time at which transition will be completed. *Treloar* presented a mathematical regression as a basis for the evaluation of the likely terminal amenorrhoea fairly representative of Caucasian women in general (Figure 2). The earliest natural menopause observed in *Treloar's* study was at 41 years, the latest at 59 years.

Improved biostatistical prediction of the time of menopause has important clinical implications; it allows one to be more appropriately aware of risk factors of diseases such as breast and endometrial cancer, enables one to give better advice regarding contraceptive methods, and provides additional information when one is trying to decide for or against ablative surgery.

A PRE-MENOPAUSAL SYNDROME?

Does the disruption of the ovulatory mechanisms and the imbalance between progesterone and oestrogen establish a characteristic syndrome of the pre-menopause? According to *Lauritzen*, around 27% of women of

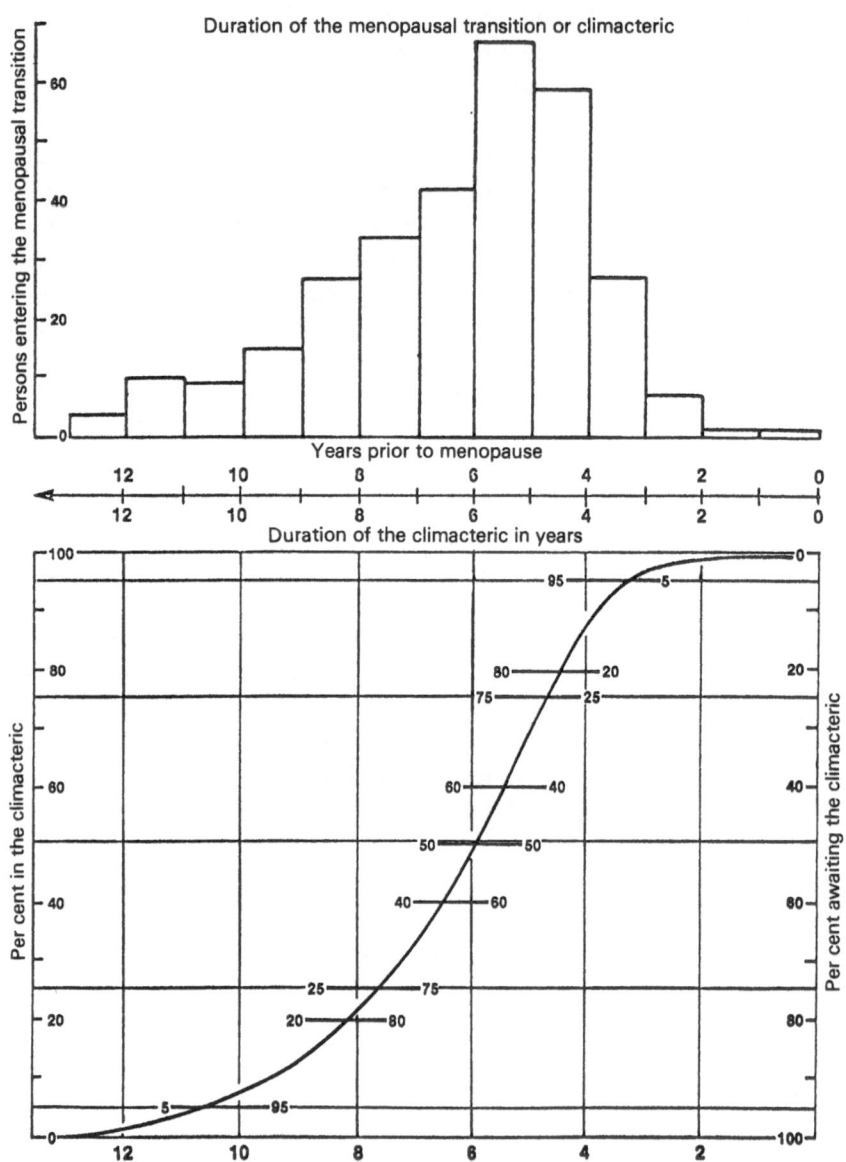

Figure 2 Normal distribution for the duration of the menopausal transition

pre-menopausal age suffer from the pre-menstrual syndrome with its typical tension, depressive mood and irritability (Table 1). These

Table 1 Principal disorders in a group of 689 pre-menopausal women attending the Universitäts-Frauen-klinik in Ulm, West Germany

Principal disorders	%
Hypermenorrhoea	11
Menorrhagia	6
Metrorrhagia	3
Pre-menstrual spotting	3
Oligomenorrhoea	17
Polymenorrhoea	13
Fibromyomata	20
Adenomyosis	3
Pre-menstrual syndrome	27
Mastopathia	26

symptoms have a considerable input from the woman's personality, which in turn is affected by her surroundings. The individual's stress may exaggerate an inherent biochemical change. To relate 'neuroticism' to these women, when their problem is brought about by metabolic changes, seems unhelpful with respect to aetiology. Of the other prevailing disorders reported by pre-menopausal women, such as sweating, a certain amount of hot flushes, dizziness, tingling sensations in the extremities, headaches, sleeplessness, worry, and anxiety (Table 2), none was found specifically to constitute a pre-menopausal syndrome. The principal worries of the pre-menopausal women about whom *Lauritzen* spoke are listed in Table 3.

ENDOMETRIAL DISEASE

The relative oestrogen dominance at pre-menopausal age is responsible for a higher than usual incidence of unscheduled bleeding, which raises the question of proper clinical management. *Whitehead* presented some data from the general screening programme of King's College Hospital in London, in which biopsies have been obtained from 317 non-oestrogen treated peri- and post-menopausal women attending a menopausal clinic; their ages ranged from 40 to 64 years. The samples were taken either with a Vabra Suction Curette or by normal dilatation and

Table 2   Incidence of complaints at various stages of the climacteric experience, as reported by women attending the Universitäts-Frauenklinik in Ulm, West Germany

Symptoms	Pre-menopause % (n=689)	Peri-menopause % (n=447)	Post-menopause	
			1–3 years % (n=131)	> 3 years % (n=219)
Hot flushes	36	69	74	42
Sweating	28	58	67	31
Dizziness	14	33	41	25
Tingling sensation in the extremities	8	20	28	11
Depressive mood	25	72	76	38
'Nervousness'	67	51	48	22
Irritability	65	49	46	17
Tenseness	44	40	33	25
Headaches	41	31	15	11
Sleeplessness	53	56	63	41
Worry	55	55	50	34
Anxiety	33	44	26	12

Table 3   Principal worries of a group of 689 pre-menopausal women attending the Universitäts-Frauenklinik in Ulm, West Germany

Principal Worries	%
Anxiety about cancer and other severe diseases	78
Climacteric complaints	15
Deterioration of relationship with husband	24
Family troubles	
Death of parents	32
Children leaving home	25
Others	16
Decrease in libido	20
Loss of energy	12
Loss of memory and of ability to concentrate	4

curettage. The endometrial histology was then correlated with the pattern of vaginal bleeding. Cystic hyperplasia was defined as simple cystic glandular change, whereas atypical hyperplasia was only diagnosed if nuclear atypia, gland reduplication and 'back-to-back' gland formation were all present.

In 178 peri-menopausal women (mean age 49.6 years), proliferative endometrium was the most common histology, being diagnosed in 59 patients (33%). Sixteen patients (9%) had cystic hyperplasia, two (1%) atypical hyperplasia, and one endometrial carcinoma.

The most common diagnosis in the post-menopausal group (139 women with a mean age of 57.2 years) was atrophic endometrium (112 patients, 80%). Cystic hyperplasia was diagnosed in three patients (2%), atypical hyperplasia in one patient (1%) and endometrial carcinoma in two patients.

As far as the bleeding patterns of patients with abnormal histology in the peri-menopausal group were concerned, almost half (8 of 19 patients) with endometrial pathology had not experienced abnormal bleeding. In the post-menopausal group, 4 of the 6 patients with abnormal histology had not bled.

These data clearly show that a significant sub-group of peri- and post-menopausal women have endometrial abnormalities which may be clinically silent, abnormal bleeding not occurring. *Whitehead* believes that these women are probably at an increased risk of the later development of endometrial carcinoma, as hyperplasia, especially the atypical form, is a well-recognized precursor of neoplasia. Additional oestrogenic stimulation in this high-risk group, in the form of oestrogen therapy, is likely to accelerate the development of neoplasia. The relatively high incidence rates of endometrial carcinoma observed soon after the start of unopposed oestrogen therapy can probably be explained by this mechanism. *Whitehead* is therefore adamant that unopposed oestrogen treatment should only be prescribed after a biopsy has been performed and endometrial pathology excluded. The availability of modern non-metal curettes makes this a simple procedure which can be done on an out-patient basis. This proposal found much support from other speakers at this workshop.

BREAST DISEASE

When considering the specific health hazards faced by women in the pre-menopause, mention must be made of breast lesions. It is known that the cervical cancer risk is already decreasing by this age, but that of breast cancer is certainly not.

Hendriks described a breast cancer screening project which is currently being conducted by the University of Nijmegen in Holland. This programme, which began in 1975, is open to all women between the ages of 35 and 65. The scheme is government-supported; the costs are approximately 40 Dutch guilders (less than $20) per woman per screening, to which the woman herself is asked to contribute 2.50 guilders (about $1). The screening is performed by mammography, and a single view is taken of each breast. Physical examinations are not carried out, but the women receive instruction in self-examination of the breasts. The total procedure takes only fifteen minutes, and it is repeated at intervals of two years. The mean X-ray dose to glandular tissue is 0.066 rad, which does not constitute a radiation danger. Suspected breast cancer cases are referred to hospital for investigation.

The study is currently at the stage of the third screening; this screening being in progress, the figures given for it must be regarded as provisional. A total of 25 920 women participated in the first screening, 17 288 in the second, and, to date, 12 721 in the third. Hospital referral rates have been 1.3%, 0.9%, and 0.7% respectively, and biopsies have been performed in 1%, 0.6%, and 0.5% of all cases. Mammary cancer was found in 0.5% of all cases at the first screening, in 0.3% at the second, and, to date, in 0.2% at the third. Six cases of breast cancer have been detected in the intervals between the programme's official examinations.

It is felt that this programme will have to continue for another three to five years before its value can really be assessed, but the results at the present stage appear to provide good arguments in favour of this sort of mass screening programme as a critical step forward in the fight against breast cancer at the first peak of risk, i.e., during the pre-menopause.

HORMONE REPLACEMENT THERAPY DURING THE PRE-MENOPAUSE

Certain pre-menopausal problems, particularly pre-menstrual ones such as mastodynia, cyclic oedema, and headaches, often call for the correction of a hormonal disequilibrium. *Sitruk-Ware* reported on her experience in administering natural progesterone to pre-menopausal women suffering such complaints, who also have low plasma levels of progesterone. She has found that 200 mg/day micronized progesterone, taken orally, can increase plasma progesterone levels to between 15 and 20 ng/ml at the third hour after administration and to between 6 and 8 ng/ml at the eighth hour. When given on days 17 to 26 of the cycle for four consecutive months, to twelve pre-menopausal women with extremely low endogenous progesterone secretion (average plasma progesterone levels of 4.5 ng/ml on days 20 to 24 of the cycle), it was found that this dose of micronized progesterone completely corrected bleeding irregularities, pre-menstrual tension, and dysmenorrhoea; mastodynia and cyclic oedema also improved in almost all cases. Body weight, blood pressure, and plasma HDL-cholesterol remained unaltered, while triglycerides were significantly lowered, from 57 ± 8 mg/dl before treatment to 41 ± 3 mg/dl after treatment, $p < 0.005$. No effect was seen on oral glucose tolerance. A minor side effect was drowsiness, which was reported by two women after a morning dose (plasma progesterone levels in these cases were 49 and 52 ng/ml).

It seems from *Sitruk-Ware*'s study that a micronized progesterone can indeed be effective in correcting luteal phase deficiencies of progesterone during the pre-menopause; the micronized preparation seems to be devoid of the metabolic side effects sometimes seen with norethisterone derivatives.

CONTRACEPTION IN THE PRE-MENOPAUSE

Pre-menopausal women tend to want to avoid pregnancy. It must be said that there are certainly good and well-known reasons from the medical standpoint as to why they should. *Notelovitz* pointed out that because of this there is usually a period of ten to fifteen years prior to the menopause during which a particularly reliable method of contraception is needed.

Reports of an increased incidence of potentially fatal conditions, such as venous thrombosis and pulmonary embolism, cardiovascular disease, coronary artery disease, and hypertension, in women over the age of 35 have, certainly in the past, made many physicians reluctant to prescribe oral contraceptives for women in this age group. Recent analyses have tended to suggest that these risks were somewhat exaggerated, at least once the lower dose preparations became available.

Notelovitz's investigations have led him to the conclusion that, provided patients are adequately screened, today's oral contraceptives, especially those containing only $30-35$ μg ethinyloestradiol and 0.4 mg of norethisterone or one of the other newer progestogens, can safely be given to women up to the age of 45. Between 45 and 50, he feels that consideration should be given to the use of an IUD, preferably of the medicated variety, and from 50 until one year after the last natural menstrual bleeding, it is his opinion that barrier methods, such as the diaphragm, condom and spermicidal jellies, should be recommended. It is also his feeling that couples who have completed their families should be encouraged, once the woman reaches pre-menopausal age, to consider sterilization, either tubal interruption or vasectomy.

CONCLUDING REMARKS

As this workshop developed it became clear that although there is no evidence at the present time of a 'pre-menopause syndrome' as such, there are certain aspects and problems which do affect women at this particular phase of life. By obtaining better insight into these, women will clearly be helped through this transitional phase, and probably also through the more problematical peri-menopause and post-menopause phases which are to follow. On reflection, it was a pity that during this workshop there was not time to dwell on the points which Professor Lauritzen has found to be those about which women are most worried at this time of life. I should like to suggest that this is an aspect to which consideration be given in the future, and which might, perhaps, be reported upon at the next congress in this series.

Reference

Treloar, A. E., Boynton, R. E., Behn, B. G. and Brown, B. W. (1967). Variation of the human menstrual cycle through reproductive life. *Int. J. Fertil.*, **12**, 77

Workshop 3

Sociological aspects of mid-life

Moderator: **M. Hepworth** (UK)

Speakers: **A. Collin** (UK)
             E. Fairhurst (UK)
             M. Featherstone (UK)
             L. Goldie (UK)
             M. Hepworth (UK)
             A. Holte (Norway)
             A. Mikkelsen (Norway)
             B. Moore (UK)
             H. Roberts (UK)
             J. Wilbush (Canada)

INTRODUCTION

Previous conferences of the International Menopause Society concluded that climacteric symptoms and complaints are the product of an inter-action between sociocultural, psychological and physical factors: "The psycho-social aspects of the menopause form an integral part of the picture and it is therefore misleading to look at the menopause and climacteric phase as purely biological phenomena" (van Keep and Humphrey, 1976). It was also agreed that the processes of interaction between social, psychological and physical factors were extremely com-plex and required much further study.

The aim of this workshop, therefore, was to bring together sociologists, psychologists and medical researchers who are seeking to interpret the particular symptoms of the menopause in terms of the cultures in which

19

they are expressed and of the everyday experiences of samples of women concerned.

In essence the workshop was in two parts, the underlying theme being continuity and change. The first part concentrated specifically on the climacteric syndrome and the menopause, and the second part examined the broader issues of changing attitudes to middle age within which contemporary discussions of the menopause can be located.

CLIMACTERIC EXPRESSION AND SOCIAL CONTEXT

In his discussion of women in Zulu and Palestinian Arab societies *Wilbush* showed how their social status depends almost entirely on the number and position of children, particularly sons, to which they have naturally given birth. A barren woman is said to be 'nothing', she is biologically and socially worthless. Similarly, a woman who becomes sterile, ceases to bear children, or reaches the climacteric, loses her biological and therefore social value. Yet despite this stressful situation and despite the physiological change of the menopause common to all middle-aged women, Zulu and Arab Palestinian women do not display the 'classical' climacteric syndrome so common in the West. Unlike their western sisters they do not regard the climacteric as an illness. The reasons for this difference in attitude can be found in the particular cultures to which they belong. Whilst women who have lost their ability to bear children also face loss of status and therefore experience considerable stress during the climacteric, they are also provided with a number of solutions to their problems which determine the ways in which they experience and communicate their change of life to others. Once beyond child-bearing years, they may firstly, acquire social children through a surrogate 'womb'; secondly, they may discover they have an important role to play in being worthless. Women who are disposable can, for example, face danger, disease, and evil spirits without fear, for no-one would bother to harm them. Thirdly, where menstrual blood is considered unclean, climacteric women can assume a special ritual status, and fourthly, they may seek to influence their husbands through the manipulation of his choice of a younger second wife.

Wilbush concluded that

the expression of climacteric stress, like any other communication, needs a 'code' in which to transmit its message. The West has evolved a code which equates social injustice with physical injury. The cultures here considered have created a code of action which makes it possible for a woman to gain mature female status despite the disadvantages of being barren.

One aspect of the peculiar nature of the western code for climacteric expression was highlighted in *Holte* and *Mikkelsen*'s study of the influence of cultural myths on climacteric reactions in a small rural area in Norway. As a result of semi-structured interviews with 61 randomly chosen women aged 45–60, a widespread myth concerning the climacteric was discovered. Its gloomy prediction was that as a consequence of hormonal changes most women could expect to experience severe physical and psychological distress; in other words, to suffer ill-health. The main sources of this myth did not appear to be direct personal experience (when asked to compare their earlier expectations with actual experiences of the change, one half of the sample said it had been better than expected and less than a third said their fears were realized), but was derived from books, weekly magazines and medical practitioners. *Holte* and *Mikkelsen* concluded that the function of the myth is to provide women with an interpretive framework within which meaning can be given to unspecific altered bodily states during the climacteric, and some assessment of personal experience made. In particular the myth appears to have an important influence on the *anticipation* of the menopause if not its realization.

On the question of the specific climacteric symptoms reported by women when questioned by medical personnel, interesting comparative data were provided in *Moore*'s analysis of 50 middle-aged women from the villages surrounding the township of Triangle in southeast Zimbabwe (Moore, 1981). The women were randomly selected and all were more than 1 and less than 10 years past the date of their last menstrual period. None had any history of gynaecological problems or had undergone any operation, and none had received any form of treatment for relief of symptoms since the menopause. None of the women spoke English or knew her exact age. Each woman was interviewed in private by a bilingual nursing sister at the hospital.

The results, recorded on a questionnaire, showed that 43% of the group reported hot flushes, sweats, palpitations, and dyspepsia in some degree and 52% reported 'psychogenic' symptoms such as insomnia, depression, and fear of ageing. In addition, 52% reported 'metabolic' symptoms such as vaginal dryness, hair or skin changes, headache and backache. Moore concluded that the incidence of climacteric symptoms in the study group was broadly similar to that recorded in a selection of surveys in western societies (e.g. Thompson *et al.*, 1973; Prill, 1977) and his research "provided no support for the popularly expressed opinion that the 'climacteric syndrome' is restricted to affluent societies in which healthy middle-aged women have the time to over-react to the loss of their youth and to the prospect of coming old age".

DOCTORS AND PATIENTS

The history of climacteric expression in the West is the history of a tension between the social origins of many of the stresses women experience in middle age and the tendency of the medical profession to locate such difficulties within changes taking place in the physical organism. Drawing on professional texts on the menopause, and a study of 300 middle-aged women and their general practitioners carried out in the UK between 1976 and 1980, *Roberts* argued that middle-aged women and their doctors have a qualitatively different way of looking at the nature, context and management of the menopause. Her concern was not with osteoporosis or vasomotor disturbances where doctors' views may carry a particular authority, but with the social construction of issues around the menopause which are as important to women as any physical discomfort or unease.

Differences in gender, social background and training have produced barriers to free communication which are all too rarely breached. Because of the social distance separating women from their doctors the former are often unwilling to reveal the full details of their personal and social problems in middle life whilst the latter rely far too heavily on the stereotype of the 'difficult' plaintive, and over-anxious 'menopausal woman' whose problems are basically physical or merely psychosomatic. The result is a kind of conspiracy between doctor and patient to agree on a description of the menopause which makes inadequate distinctions between 'real' symptoms which a doctor can treat and 'vague' symptoms which do not warrant treatment. At the same time *Roberts*'s research confirms that women place a high value on doctors with whom they can discuss their problems sympathetically and therefore it is all the more important for the medical profession to become better versed in the realities of the everyday lives of their patients.

One of the problems facing a woman during the climacteric is to decide whether she is experiencing a 'normal' or an 'abnormal' menopause. The paper presented by *Fairhurst* reported a study in the UK (Fairhurst and Lightup, 1980) involving in-depth interviews with 18 women attending a menopause clinic at a hospital and two groups comprising 16 'well women' who were approached via the age–sex register of two general practitioners. The general practices were located in a working-class and middle-class area. In addition, interviews were carried out with 24 men. All interviewees were married and the women were aged 50 (according to Gray, 1976, the modal age of menopause) in the year the research began.

The results indicate that women interpret their physical and psychological feelings by means of a complex process of self-assessment. *Fairhurst* stressed that it was essential to recognize that these women measured normality in terms of their own notion of what was normal for them (their self-concept) against their ideas, derived from discussions with family, friends, and some reading, of what was normal for all women going through the menopause. When this self-assessment ran contrary to their personal concept of the normal, medical advice would be sought. Thus the sample of 'well-women' had decided that their feelings were not out of the ordinary and did not merit recourse to the medical profession, yet the sample attending the menopause clinic had decided that their feelings (which were not, it is important to note, necessarily different from those of the 'well women') were not acceptable to them. *Fairhurst*'s general conclusion, which confirms *Roberts*'s findings, was that symptoms presented to a doctor are thus of limited value in understanding women's experience of the menopause: greater understanding depends on deeper inside knowledge of the personal meaning of these symptoms to the woman concerned.

Further evidence of the depth and complexity of the emotional problems which can beset women at mid-life was provided in *Goldie*'s discussion of case histories of patients who had received psychotherapy in the UK. In confirmation of previous sociological studies (*Roberts* and *Fairhurst*), he noted that many of the difficulties of which menopausal women complain are mistakenly attributed to the age and physical condition of the patient. All the anxieties of the 'menopause' – a sense of failure, a feeling that time is running out, the loss of athleticism, the idea that one is old and finished, diminishing sexual potency, loneliness and isolation – can be seen in other age groups. The menopause is, in effect, a coincidence of many crises. In this sense it is mythical: the associated problems are not biological in origin but stem from the patient's personal situation and resources for coming to terms with an altered state.

Long before the menopause a woman may become acutely conscious of the passage of time and the realization that life is unrepeatable: that ageing is inexorable. Child-bearing may have served to justify her existence or to compensate, for example, for feelings of inadequacy as a sexual partner. After the menopause such supports and compensations are no longer viable and she must find alternative solutions to her problem.

One solution, as *Wilbush* also intimated, is to seek medical advice. Not infrequently, *Goldie* observed, the doctor feels he is under pressure from a menopausal patient to wave a magic wand in the form of drugs or HRT which will hopefully banish distress and even recapture lost youth: 'the good old days' that were or could have been. But undue reliance on chemotherapy derives from the belief that chemical changes must account for all mental changes and there is no need to be dependent on them. The patient thus tends to become passive, taking a drug on advice, and thereby submitting to a constraint on her activities and feelings.

Because it is the pre-menopausal personality and culture rather than endocrine changes which determine emotional reactions during the climacteric, the experience of physical change merely emphasizes and revives long-standing fears of ageing, impotence, and death. The personal interpretation of symptoms, as *Fairhurst* indicated, is of paramount importance. Chemotherapy should therefore be used sparingly in order not to undermine a patient's capacity to face up to the reality of her personal and social problems and to make decisions about the future. In practice good advice and psychotherapy are aimed to activate and sponsor the patient's independence and mobilize her depression so she can realize her neglected creativity and the opportunities for future positive personal change.

CHANGE IN MIDDLE AGE AND CHANGING ATTITUDES TO MIDDLE AGE

Unlike the preceding contributions to the workshop, *Collin*'s discussion of the 'mid-life crisis' concentrated for the most part on the male experience of middle age. She presented a review of clinical case histories, cross-sectional analyses, and longitudinal studies which argue that there is evidence of a transitional stage in male middle age analogous to the physical and emotional crisis of the menopause. This crisis is popularly described as the 'male menopause' or more commonly the 'mid-life crisis'.

In the academic literature (in USA, UK, France and Germany) the 'mid-life crisis' represents the epitome of change in the middle-aged male, the nodal points being:

(1) response to physical ageing (changing body-image and self-image, diminishing sex drive);
(2) resurgence of repressed/suppressed instincts (rebalancing id/ego creativity);
(3) awareness of personal mortality (changed perception of time, aspiration–achievement gap, a search for new goals);
(4) rôle changes (rôle losses, rôle asynchronization, intergenerational problems);
(5) crisis: generativity versus stagnation.

These changes can take place over an extended period from around the age of 35 onwards and can be far-reaching and often painful. The debate, however, about whether these changes may typically be seen as a syndrome experienced by all men during the middle years, and whether the symptoms may meaningfully be interpreted as those of a mid-life crisis, continues between popular literature and academic researcher. The main issue thus hinges upon the question *specificity* versus *universality*.

Collin's provisional conclusion is that although sociological and psychological research into middle age is in its infancy, there is at present little evidence to support the universality thesis. On the other hand, there can be little doubt that the attitudes of men and of women towards middle age are being modified in response to sociocultural change. The concept of middle age is itself going through a transitional stage: we are witnessing, she suggests, the death throes of the conventional stereotype of middle age as the end of youthful energy, body-imagery and outlook. The concept of the 'mid-life crisis' has caught the public imagination because the current generation of middle-aged is finding this period of life not at all what they expected. Their unease and disquiet at having to grapple with unexpected problems, where traditional rôle models of middle-aged stability and confidence are becoming outmoded, has coalesced around the notion of 'mid-life crisis'. It has the advantage in an ambiguous situation of providing some explanation of their feelings, anxieties, and fears, and when necessary provides a justification for certain kinds of behaviour which might otherwise be considered deviant.

Confirmatory evidence of the changing expectations of men and women with regard to middle age was offered in the final discussion of this workshop by *Featherstone* and *Hepworth* on changing images of middle age. Their study involved the analysis of treatments of the menopause, the 'male menopause', the 'mid-life crisis', and middle age, in the press, television, cinema, advertising, popular fiction, and psychological and sociological publications in the UK between 1972 and 1980.

This analysis of popular culture shows that a new vocabulary of middle age is emerging: a new resource for the identification, description, and solution of problems in mid-life is replacing the old language of resignation and acceptance of the imminence of old age. Such a language is encapsulated in the new image of middle age which emphasizes the value of a youthful appearance and presentation of self earned through care for one's health, efforts to maintain physical fitness, and the constant pursuit of longevity. The rewards for these efforts are said to be an enhanced lifestyle and the greater assurance of happiness and an anxiety-free existence, and members of all social classes are now under pressure from a wide variety of interests to struggle against the physical signs of ageing. Those who allow their health and therefore appearance to deteriorate are running the risk of being identified as failures, for in western society, as many other commentators have noted (Henry, 1963), decrepit old age is synonymous with personal failure.

The new image of middle age has its positive and negative aspects. On the negative side there are all the anxieties and fears associated with the menopause, the 'male menopause' and the 'mid-life crisis' *(Goldie, Collin)*. On the positive side can be found an increasing number of popular and academic publications (cf. *Collin*) describing the middle years as a new and challenging period of life totally different in lifestyle and quality from the middle age of a generation past; that is, those who are now in what Henry (1963) described as 'deep old age'.

Thus the image sensitizes the middle-aged to the problems they can and sometimes ought to expect in the middle years and simultaneously offers a number of solutions to these difficulties, all of which centre around the possibility of rejuvenation and personal change. Because this movement shows no sign of deceleration it is expected that the quality of life in middle age, as well as the problems associated with it, will be significantly different for the present and later generations than was the case in the past.

CONCLUSIONS

On the basis of detailed analyses of specific cultures and the meanings given to the menopause in those cultures, small-scale qualitative studies involving in-depth interviews with samples of female and male subjects, clinical case histories, and surveys of the academic literature, this workshop arrived at the following conclusions.

(1) The menopause is not an independent variable but a social construct, the meaning of which is created and sustained through processes of human communication.

(2) Studies of other cultures show that illness (i.e. the reporting of menopausal symptoms to a doctor) is not the only possible reaction to the kinds of stress women experience during middle age; differring cultures provide women with varying vocabularies, tactics, and resources for handling stress in middle age.

(3) Following from the above, it is important, if greater understanding of middle age and the menopause is required, to study:

    (i) the ways in which women assign meaning to middle age in general and to the menopause in particular. Here there are two questions for which a woman must find answers: (a) What is a 'normal' menopause? (b) How can I tell if my menopause is abnormal?

    (ii) It is also therefore necessary to study the kinds of advice available to women before they consult the medical profession and the factors influencing any decision to seek a doctor's help.

(4) Small-scale studies in the UK suggest that female patients and their doctors tend at present to use the stereotype of the typical 'menopausal woman' who is over-anxious about physical change, as a main vehicle for communication. Despite the fact that many of the problems of women during climacteric reflect their particular situation and rôle, these difficulties tend to be pushed aside in favour of a purely organic approach. This puts serious limitations on our knowledge of the menopause.

(5) Western attitudes to middle age amongst women and men are gradually changing in response to pressures from health education, preventive medicine, and from the mass media, and consumer culture. These changes are often labelled the 'mid-life crisis' and sometimes the 'male menopause'. There are signs that a new lifestyle is being created by and for the middle-aged, placing great value on youth, fitness and active sexuality.

(6) The above changes have important implications for the menopause because they encourage a new consciousness of the ageing body

which was less apparent amongst the middle-aged of past generations. Consequently there is likely to be an increasing demand for preparations, services and advice to enable both women and men to remain physically and sexually active in later life.

References

Collin, A. (1979). 'Mid-life crisis' and its implications in counselling. *Br. J. Guid. Counsel.*, **7**, 144

Fairhurst, E. and Lightup, R. (1980). Being menopausal: women and medical treatment. Paper presented to the Medical Sociology Group Conference of the British Sociological Association, University of Warwick

Featherstone, M. and Hepworth, M. (1980). Changing images of middle age. In Johnson, M. L. (ed.) *Transitions in Middle and Later Life*. (London: British Society of Gerontology)

Gray, R. H. (1976). The menopause – epidemiological and demographic considerations. In Beard, R. J. (ed.) *The Menopause: A Guide to Current Research and Practice*. (Baltimore: University Park Press)

Henry, J. (1963). *Culture Against Man*. (New York: Random House)

van Keep, P. A. and Humphrey M. (1976). Psycho-social aspects of the climacteric. In van Keep, P. A., Greenblatt, R. B. and Albeaux-Fernet, M. (eds.) *Consensus On Menopause Research*. (Lancaster: MTP Press)

Moore, B. (1981). Climacteric symptoms in an African community. *Maturitas, 3*, 1

Prill, H. J. (1977). A study of the socio-medical relationships at the climacteric in 2232 women. *Curr. Med. Res. Opin.*, **4**, (Suppl.) 3

Thompson, B., Hart, S. A. and Durno, D. (1973). Menopausal age and symptomatology in a general practice. *J. Biosocial Sci.*, **5**, 71

Workshop 4

Some biochemical consequences of post-menopausal hormone replacement treatment

Moderator: **U. Larsson-Cohn** (Sweden)

Speakers: **M. G. Crane** (USA)
L. Fåhraeus (Sweden)
E. Hirvonen (Finland)
U. Larsson-Cohn (Sweden)
M. A. Limouzin-Lamothe (France)
M. Notelovitz (USA)
B. von Schoultz (Sweden)
J. W. W. Studd (UK)

INTRODUCTION

In 1976 during the First International Congress on the Menopause, I (*Larsson-Cohn*) had the pleasure of chairing a workshop with a title similar to that of the present one. On that occasion it became clear that until the mid-seventies very little investigative work had been done on the metabolic consequences of post-menopausal hormone replacement therapy. Some studies had been performed in connection with the effects of combined oral contraceptive agents, but it was difficult to extrapolate from these the effects of oestrogens *per se*, and those of progestogens. The problem was further complicated by the fact that at that time it was not unusual for authors to state merely that the women in their studies had been taking 'oral contraceptives', without specifying the composition of the preparations taken. In other instances the results from subjects taking different oral contraceptive agents were pooled.

Today, although our knowledge is still far from complete, it is clear that we have a better understanding of this subject than we had six years ago.

This report on the workshop over which I presided at the Third International Congress on the Menopause deals mainly with the influence of exogenous sexual steroids on blood pressure, on lipid and carbohydrate metabolism, and on liver function, with special emphasis on lipids and lipoproteins.

Regrettably, many investigators attempt to compare the biochemical and hormonal effects of different oestrogenic drugs without carefully considering if equipotent doses are used; for this reason the workshop began with a presentation by *von Schoultz* in which he discussed the various methods used to quantify oestrogenicity. The next three presentations, by myself, by *Fåhraeus*, and by *Hirvonen*, dealt with the effects of post-menopausal hormone replacement therapy on plasma lipids and lipoproteins. *Notelovitz* then discussed oestrogen therapy and carbohydrate metabolism, and *Studd* briefly reported on the effects, or rather on the lack of effects, of oestradiol + testosterone implants on the liver. The final two speakers were *Crane* and *Limouzin-Lamothe*, who spoke on the effects of post-menopausal oestrogen therapy on hypertension.

METHODS TO QUANTIFY OESTROGENICITY (Introduced by B. von Schoultz)

A great many parameters are used to 'quantify' oestrogenicity, but the value of these differs considerably with regard to sensitivity and to clinical relevance.

One might consider that an assessment based on the proliferation of the endometrium and/or the vaginal epithelium would be valid, since improvements here would certainly reflect increased oestrogenicity. The problem with this as a parameter is that clinically the response is difficult to quantify, and the assays available at present are not able to differentiate well between the effects of different treatments. Theoretically, human *in vivo* studies of receptor affinity, or quantitative assays of progesterone receptor induction in target organs, would seem ideal ways of quantifying oestrogenic potency, but for the moment these approaches are hampered by technical problems. Good assays *are* available for measuring the inhibition of gonadotrophins, and these do indeed reveal differences between therapies. However, for this method to be of real value one must be sure of the correlation between a certain reduction in circulating gonadotrophins and particular therapeutic effects or unwanted side effects.

Among the many biochemical effects seen following oestrogen therapy, one of the most interesting is the increase in liver protein synthesis. Assays for measuring oestrogen-induced plasma proteins, SHBG (sex hormone binding globulin), CBG (cortisol binding globulin), and ceruloplasmin, for example, are very sensitive and reveal dose-dependent patterns during therapy. This approach offers several advantages, as the changes seen reflect an 'efferent' expression of steroid influence. Thus the net oestrogenic effect, which can easily be monitored by serial measurements in patient serum, allows for variations in intestinal absorption, protein binding, and intracellular metabolism.

LIPIDS AND LIPOPROTEINS (Introduced by U. Larsson-Cohn)

In Western societies mortality in CVD (cardiovascular disease) is much higher in 40–50-year-old males than it is in females of a similar age. It has been known for some time that plasma concentrations of cholesterol and of triglycerides are directly correlated with the risk of CVD, but it has recently become evident that the lipoprotein pattern is of greater significance in this context. In some situations the total plasma cholesterol may remain unchanged, while the cholesterol within the HDL (high density lipoprotein) fraction, the 'good cholesterol', is altered significantly. Women have higher plasma concentrations of HDL than men, and experimental and epidemiological studies have shown that low HDL-cholesterol levels and/or high LDL (low density lipoprotein)-cholesterol levels are potent risk factors for CVD (Gordon *et al.*, 1977; Steinberg, 1978). There are two major HDL subfractions, HDL_2 and HDL_3, and it is believed that it is the HDL_2, subfraction which is associated with the lowered CVD risk.

Untreated premature menopause is associated with raised CVD morbidity and mortality (Johansson *et al.*, 1975; Hammond *et al.*, 1979; Rosenberg *et al.*, 1981), and recently Ross *et al.* (1981) have reported that post-menopausal women who have taken oestrogens for many years have a mortality rate in ischaemic heart disease which is 50% lower than that of controls. Thus there are now epidemiological data suggesting that women under oestrogen influence, either from endogenous or exogenous sources, have a lower cardiovascular morbidity and mortality than those deprived of this hormonal stimulation.

31

The next two reports, those of *Fåhraeus* and of *Hirvonen*, confirm earlier studies which showed that post-menopausal oestrogen therapy induces changes in the lipoprotein pattern which are believed to be anti-atherogenic. This is, of course, a strong corroboration of the suggestion that oestrogen therapy may reduce the cardiovascular disease risk.

EFFECTS OF POST-MENOPAUSAL HORMONE REPLACEMENT THERAPIES ON LIPIDS AND LIPOPROTEINS (Introduced by L. Fåhraeus)

There were two parts to this study. In the first, 38 post-menopausal women still experiencing climacteric symptoms were each randomly assigned to one of two types of cyclical oestradiol treatment: one group received oral oestradiol, 2 mg/day for four months, followed by 4 mg/day for two months, while the other received 3 mg/day percutaneous oestradiol. The two treatments were evaluated after six cycles.

In both groups plasma oestrone and oestradiol increased significantly, while FSH (follicle stimulating hormone) and LH (luteinizing hormone) decreased significantly. Percutaneous oestradiol induced only small lipid changes, while the oral treatment decreased LDL and increased HDL significantly, the latter mainly due to rises in HDL_2 levels. The higher dose of oral oestradiol (4 mg/day) increased triglycerides. In contrast to the oral oestradiol, the percutaneous oestradiol did not induce a high post-medication plasma oestrogen peak, and, of course, reached the peripheral circulation without first passing the enterohepatic circulation. These differences probably lead to a less pronounced induction of the various liver enzymes. The differences in the effects on lipid metabolism between the two oestradiol treatments may probably be explained by these variations in the pharmakinetic behaviour of the two drugs.

In the second part of the study, 24 women who had received percutaneous oestradiol for 4–6 months were additionally given either 120 μg levon ·estrel/day or 300 mg progesterone/day for the last eleven days of a further six cycles of percutaneous oestradiol. In the women receiving oestradiol + levonorgestrel there was a pronounced lowering of HDL, accounted for mainly by a reduction in the HDL_2 concentration, but in the women receiving oestradiol + progesterone only small, non-significant, lipoprotein changes occurred.

The results of this study are summarized in Figure 1. The conclusion from it is that in order to avoid unwanted effects on lipid metabolism during post-menopausal oestrogen + progestogen medication, it is essential to balance the effects of the two components. This also applies, of course, to oestrogen + progestogen oral contraceptive use (Larsson-Cohn et al., 1981). From the lipoprotein point of view, it would seem that androgenic testosterone derived progestogens should probably be avoided, or given only in low dosages.

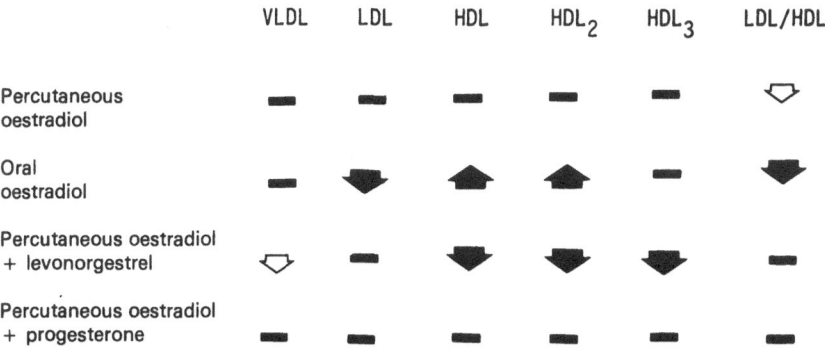

Figure 1 Summary of the effects of the post-menopausal administration of various hormone replacement therapies on lipids and lipoproteins. The black arrows indicate statistically significant changes in the major lipid components on at least two of the three sampling occasions, the white arrows indicate a statistically significant change either in two major lipid components on one sampling occasion or in one lipid component on two occasions, and the dashes indicate no change. (Reproduced by kind permission of L. Fåhraeus)

The recent report from Ross et al. (1981) indicating that post-menopausal oral oestrogen therapy has a protective effect against death from ischaemic heart disease, leads to the conclusion that the changes seen in this study when oral oestradiol was given (see Figure 1) should be regarded as beneficial ones.

EFFECTS OF PROGESTOGENS ON LIPOPROTEINS DURING POST-MENOPAUSAL REPLACEMENT THERAPY (Introduced by E. Hirvonen)

It is clear that during treatment with oestrogen + progestogen combinations the effects on lipoprotein metabolism vary depending on the dose of the oestrogen and on the oestrogenic, anti-oestrogenic, androgenic, and anti-androgenic activities of the progestogen. Progestogen derivatives of 19-nortestosterone possess some androgenic properties, but alcylated or halogenated acetoxyprogesterone derivatives do not – they are regarded as 'pure' progestogens, possessing neither oestrogenic nor androgenic properties.

In a recent study (Hirvonen *et al.*, 1981) three groups of post-menopausal women were each treated with a different sequential oestradiol + progestogen regimen. All the women received 2 mg/day oestradiol valerate for three weeks of each cycle; on days 15–24 of each cycle group A additionally received 10 mg/day norethisterone acetate, group B 10 mg/day medroxyprogesterone acetate, and group C 0.5 mg/day norgestrel. After two treatment cycles it was found that total cholesterol had decreased in all groups by 10–18% ($p < 0.05$). The difference between the various regimens was that whilst no significant change occurred in HDL-cholesterol in the women receiving medroxyprogesterone acetate, decreases of 20% were seen in the women receiving norethisterone acetate and in those receiving norgestrel ($p < 0.01$).

This suggests that the androgenic 19-nortestosterone derivatives reverse the beneficial effect of oestrogens on lipoproteins, whereas the acetoxyprogesterone derivatives, at least the medroxyprogesterone acetate tested here, do not.

OESTROGEN REPLACEMENT THERAPY AND CARBOHYDRATE METABOLISM IN PERI-MENOPAUSAL WOMEN (Introduced by M. Notelovitz)

Oestrogens probably temporarily alter glucose tolerance. This is not associated with hyperinsulinaemia, but does result in some lowering of fasting blood glucose; the adverse effects of this are usually biphasic, with elevated blood glucose levels normalizing in most instances once treatment has continued for six months or so. The hyperglycaemia may be related to dose and to potency, rather than to the *type* of oestrogen. In some subjects the disturbance persists after cessation of treatment, due to latent diabetes. Thus oestrogen therapy may be described as having a glucogenic (reversible), rather than a diabetogenic (permanent), potential.

The pathogenesis of oestrogen-mediated hyperglycaemia is undetermined; an effect on the enterohormone mechanism of early insulin release, alterations in the portal ratio of insulin:glucagon, an increase in growth hormone or in cortisol, and an ill-defined increase in the peripheral resistance to insulin, have all been incriminated.

34

Correct oestrogen usage does not generally result in significant or prolonged alterations in glucose tolerance, but some idiosyncratic responses may occur, and it is therefore recommended that a 2 h post-glucose blood glucose level be determined annually. Diabetes *per se* is not an absolute contraindication for oestrogen therapy in the peri-menopause.

LIVER FUNCTION TESTS IN WOMEN WITH OESTRADIOL + TESTOSTERONE IMPLANTS (Introduced by J. W. W. Studd)

Twenty-four women were given subcutaneous implants of 50 mg oestradiol + 100 mg testosterone every sixth month for two years. Serum bilirubin, AST, gamma-GTP, and alkaline phosphatase remained normal throughout the two-year period, as did the results of radio-isotope liver scans. It may therefore be said that no signs were found of any abnormal liver function, or of store occupying adenomata.

OESTROGENS AND HYPERTENSION (Introduced by M. G. Crane)

Oestrogens in therapeutic doses have been found to increase plasma renin substrate, plasma renin activity, aldosterone excretion, and exchangeable sodium, and to decrease plasma renin concentration. The discontinuation of oestrogen therapy has been found to result, within one month, in a significant decrease in plasma renin activity, renin substrate, aldosterone excretion, and exchangeable sodium. Renin substrate has been found to be above normal in 75% of patients one month after the discontinuation of oestrogen therapy.

Medroxyprogesterone and ethynodiol diacetate have been found to increase exchangeable sodium, to decrease aldosterone excretion, but not to change renin substrate or renin activity. Natural progesterone, on the other hand, has been found to cause a slight but significant decrease in exchangeable sodium, an increase in plasma renin activity and aldosterone excretion, but no change in renin substrate.

This appears to support the conclusion that oestrogens induce sodium retention by production of a hyperaldosterone state through their effect on renin substrate and by a direct sodium retaining effect on renal tubules. Synthetic progestational agents have a direct sodium retaining effect on the kidney. Natural progesterone, however, has an 'anti-aldosterone' sodium losing effect, but this is characteristically suppressed during oestrogen administration. The net result of the sodium retention and of other factors is that in certain susceptible individuals hypertension ensues.

Approximately half of the women who develop hypertension whilst using an oestrogenic compound may be expected to become normotensive within one year of discontinuing its use. It is also worth noting that patients usually respond well to a beta-blocker and/or a hydrochlorothiazide spironolactone preparation when the oestrogen therapy needs to be continued.

INFLUENCE OF THE ROUTE OF ADMINISTRATION OF OESTRADIOL ON ANGIOTENSINOGEN HEPATIC SYNTHESIS (Introduced by M. A. Limouzin-Lamothe)

The aim of the study reported here was to compare the effects on angiotensinogen hepatic synthesis of two different routes of administration, oral versus percutaneous, of the same natural oestrogen: oestradiol.

Twenty post-menopausal women, aged 48–72, entered the trial. All had experienced the menopause at least one year earlier, and all were suffering oestrogen-deficiency symptoms, mainly hot flushes or vulvo-vaginal atrophy.

They were first given 2 mg/day oral micronized oestradiol for one full month, then, after 10 days during which no treatment was given, they were given, again for one full month, 5 g/day percutaneous oestradiol gel, i.e. 3 mg/day oestradiol. It is estimated that some 10% of the oestrogen is absorbed through the skin. Blood samples were taken, always between 0800 and 1000 h, before treatment began, and then 2 h after the last ingestion of oral oestradiol, and 24–27 h after the last application of the percutaneous oestradiol.

From the clinical standpoint, the two treatments achieved similar effects regarding relief from oestrogen-deficiency symptoms, and were regarded as equipotent by the patients.

The one month's treatment with oral oestradiol caused a highly significant increase in angiotensinogen I. The increase varied greatly, from 20% to 300%. It was not possible to detect a correlation between the pretreatment levels and the increase in individual women. After one month's therapy with the percutaneous oestradiol the angiotensinogen I level significantly decreased in all patients, and there was a marked tendency towards normalization. The average angiotensinogen I level after the two months of treatment was not significantly different from the pretreatment level.

Blood pressure changes, either diastolic or systolic, were seen in 8 of the 20 patients during treatment. No correlation could be found between changes in the plasma renin substrate and changes in the blood pressure.

Although this study involved only a small number of patients, it is felt that several conclusions may be drawn:

(1) Plasma levels of renin substrate measured prior to hormonal therapy are of no value in predicting the risk of hypertension during oestrogen treatment.

(2) As high levels of plasma renin substrate did not appear to correlate with elevated blood pressure, the increase seen in angio-tensinogen synthesis must be regarded mainly as an effect of the oestrogen on the liver.

(3) In this connection, it is clear that 3 mg/day oestradiol given percutaneously (5 g gel) does not affect liver protein synthesis, whereas 2 mg/day of the same natural hormone given orally most certainly does.

It is likely that the difference seen in this study between the oral and the percutaneous routes of administration also affects other aspects of liver function.

References

Gordon, T., Castelli, W. P., Hjortland, M. C. and Kannel, W. B. (1977). The predic-tion of coronary heart disease by high-density and other lipoproteins; an historical perspective. In Rifkind, B. M. and Levy, R. I. (eds.) *Hyperlipidemia*, p. 71. (New York: Grune and Stratton)

Hammond, C. B., Jelovsek, F. R., Lee, K. L., Creasman, W. T. and Parker, R. T. (1979). Effects of long-term estrogen replacement therapy. I. Metabolic effects. *Am. J. Obstet. Gynecol.*, **133**, 525

Hirvonen, E., Mälkönen, M. and Manninen, V. (1981). Effects of different progest-ogens on lipoproteins during postmenopausal replacement therapy. *N. Engl. J. Med.*, **304**, 560

Johansson, M. W., Kaij, L., Kullander, S., Lennér, H.-C., Svanberg, L. and Åstedt, B. (1975). On some late effects of bilateral oophorectomy in the age range 15–30 years. *Acta Obstet. Gynecol. Scand.*, **54**, 499

Larsson-Cohn, U., Fåhraeus, L., Wallentin, L. and Zador, G. (1981). Lipoprotein changes may be minimized by proper composition of a combined oral contraceptive. *Fertil. Steril.*, **35**, 172

Rosenberg, L., Hennekens, C. H., Rosner, B., Belander, C., Rothman, K. J. and Spizer, F. E. (1981). Early menopause and the risk of myocardial infarction. *Am. J. Obstet. Gynecol.*, **139**, 47

Ross, R. K., Paganini-Hill, A., Mack, T. M., Arthur, M. and Henderson, B. E. (1981). Menopausal oestrogen therapy and protection from death from ischaemic heart disease. *Lancet*, **1**, 858

Steinberg, D. (1978). The rediscovery of high density lipoprotein; a negative risk factor in atherosclerosis. *Eur. J. Clin. Invest.*, **8**, 107

Workshop 5

Psycho-sexual aspects of mid-life

Moderators: **A. A. Haspels** (The Netherlands)
H. Musaph (The Netherlands)

Speakers: **S. Ballinger** (Australia)
F. Bottiglioni (Italy)
L. Dennerstein (Australia)
A. Holte (Norway)
R. Lax* (USA)
B. de Lignières (France)
B. Maoz (Israel)
A. Mikkelsen (Norway)
P. Sarrel (USA)
M. de Senarclens (Switzerland)

INTRODUCTION

The second half of the last decade saw the development of two rather new and distinct kinds of literature on the problems encountered by women in mid-life. One featured papers, mainly by medical people, which tended to link psycho-sexual problems, such as dryness and soreness of the vagina, dyspareunia, and decreased libido, with endocrinologically determined changes in the sexual organs (van Keep and Gregory, 1977; Lauritzen and Müller, 1977; Musaph and Haspels, 1977; Haspels and

---

*At the last minute Dr Lax was unable to be present at the congress; her paper was read by Professor Musaph.

Musaph, 1979). The other focused on the influence of psycho-social factors, on the problems encountered by the peri-menopausal woman within her family, and within her cultural setting (Flint, 1975; Maoz *et al.*, 1978).

It was pleasing to see that at this workshop the medical and the non-medical people really tried to integrate their two approaches. In particular, the medical participants showed considerable open-mindedness regarding the psycho-social aspects. This was good to see, for it is clear that although the attitude of members of the family is important in influencing the woman's menopausal experience, the attitudes and opinions of the doctor – his judgements and prejudices – are also extremely important and influential.

SEXUALITY AND THE MENOPAUSE

The first speaker was *Bottiglioni* who presented some data from a study he has made on the sexual activity of women between the ages of 40 and 65, and of how this changes with age and menopausal status, i.e., pre-menopause, peri-menopause, early post-menopause, and late post-menopause. His study was based on 756 women who sought advice for various climacteric problems at the Menopause Clinic in Bologna, Italy. These women were interviewed by a team of gynaecologists and psychologists, using a questionnaire devised by the Department of Psychology at the University of Bologna. The main parameters were: frequency of sexual intercourse, sexual satisfaction, orgasmic response, and sexual drive. The study showed that:

(1) Women are least sexually active in the late post-menopause.
(2) Greatest sexual satisfaction and the best orgasmic response seem to occur in the pre-menopause.
(3) The frequency of sexual intercourse drops rather abruptly in the early post-menopause.
(4) Sexual drive seems to be weakest in the late post-menopause.

Bottiglioni's conclusions from his study are that (a) sexual activity decreases with age, and (b) the menopause accentuates the age-related decline.

De Senarclens then described an experiment she has recently conducted with a discussion group of six female patients aged between 47 and 57. Five of the women were married and one was a widow. It is already known from psychoanalytical research that the problems which middle-aged people have to overcome are basically the same as those faced in puberty and adolescence (King, 1980). *De Senarclen*'s experiment confirmed this. In the course of the discussion sessions it became clear that behind the need for idealization there lurked a certain aggressiveness. These feelings were strongly connected with dependency/independency conflicts, just as in puberty and adolescence. Furthermore, the same problems of gender identity in making a new life after menopause, in which social functions take on a new meaning, came to the fore. Once again, as in puberty and adolescence, a reconciliation had to be made between duty and desire. 'Termination problems' are, as we know, connected with problems of overcoming loss and separation. Here too, the problems of the middle-aged are the same as those of adolescents.

Sarrel presented some basic data relating to 50 middle-aged couples who attended the Department of Obstetrics and Gynecology at Yale School of Medicine between 1976 and 1980 for counselling because of sexual dysfunction.

The average age of the women was 54, and that of the men 57. All the women were at least three years post-menopause; ten had undergone surgical menopause. None was receiving hormone replacement therapy. Thirty-three of the women were experiencing hot flushes. Fourteen reported a change in their perception of touch, i.e., they experienced feelings of 'numbness' and/or an aversion to being touched.

Thirty-eight of the men complained of secondary erectile difficulty; of these, 7 were also troubled by premature ejaculation, and 2 by ejaculatory inhibition. In 28 cases the secondary erectile difficulties had begun shortly before or within three years after the female partner's menopause; in the other 10 cases there had been a long, but intermittent, history of sexual dysfunction which had become worse around the time of the menopause.

Thirty of the female partners of men with sexual dysfunction also had sexual problems; 19 suffered from dyspareunia and 11 were non-orgasmic (3 had never had an orgasm and 8 had become anorgasmic since their menopause).

Menopausal changes had affected sexual relations both emotionally and physically. Feelings which interfered with sexual spontaneity were the most common problems. The most frequently mentioned complaints of the female partners were vaginal dryness, vaginismus, and feelings of not wanting to be touched.

Dyspareunia and erectile difficulties were simultaneously present in

19 of the couples. In 18 of these cases the women suffered vaginismus. Vaginal dryness, which was invariably present in these cases, led to feelings of rejection. When atrophic vaginitis was accompanied by bleeding, fear of hurting became a dominant and inhibitory feeling during intercourse.

Feelings of male sexual inadequacy often stemmed from the failure of the women to respond to sexual stimulation. It was felt that in six cases sexual performance anxiety on the part of the male was the cause of the sexual dysfunction.

Sarrel spoke of the physical difficulties which some patients experience with penetration, of the slowness of the sex response cycle, and of the wide range of inhibiting emotions, such as a fear of hurting, feelings of rejection, of inadequacy and of anger, which can combine to interfere with the male sexual response.

His finding of a change in sensory perception in some women – in 14 of the 50 he reported upon – is interesting. This feeling, which seems to apply to all parts of the body, is sometimes described as a feeling of 'numbness', and sometimes as a feeling of 'not wanting to be touched'. In the latter case it can be part of a general state of hyperirritability. For the male partner a woman's insensitivity to touch or her dislike of being touched is experienced as a rejection, and in *Sarrel*'s study all of the men whose wives reported having this sensory change had erectile problems. This finding corroborates an earlier report on the immense importance of the skin as a sexual organ, particularly as far as older people are concerned (Musaph, 1977).

Ballinger and *Howe* spoke about the problem of loss of libido in women around the time of the menopause. This problem was reported by 91 (70%) of 129 menopause clinic patients involved in a recent study of theirs. In this study 'loss of libido' was defined in terms of four variables:
- frequency of intercourse
- frequency of orgasm
- degree of sexual desire
- enjoyment of sexual activity.

As expected, women with loss of libido had intercourse significantly less frequently than other women. Furthermore, 75% reported a decreased orgasmic capacity, 80% experienced less desire for sexual activity (compared with only 2% of women with no change in libido), and 68% reported decreased satisfaction with sexual activity.

The following tendencies were noted in the women reporting loss of libido:

(a) They had husbands (not lovers).

(b) Their husbands sometimes suffered erectile impotence.

(c) The majority of these women said that an active sex life was important to their husbands, but approximately half did not regard it as important for themselves. Most of these women felt guilty about their loss of libido, and continued having intercourse for their husband's sakes, thereby ensuring a vicious circle in which their guilt and resentment added to their lack of desire and enjoyment.

(d) An interesting factor, and quite unrelated to the climacteric, was that women with loss of libido were significantly more likely than other women to suffer anorgasmia. These women have never received reinforcement for sexual activity in the form of orgasm, so this finding is not surprising.

(e) An unexpected finding was that dry vagina is not related to loss of libido. Surprisingly nearly twice as many women in the group with no change in libido reported vaginal dryness at intercourse. Women in the group reporting loss of libido complained not only of dryness at intercourse, but also of vaginal soreness.

(f) There was significantly more depression and anxiety in the group with loss of libido. All depressions were diagnosed as reactive depressions in this highly atypical sample.

Ballinger and *Howe* have concluded that loss of libido, at least in the women they studied, is related not only to the menopause, but also to several other factors: marital relations, life stresses, anorgasmia, and depression and anxiety. They found that only vaginal soreness bore any consistent and relationship to loss of libido.

Holte and *Mikkelsen* reported on a study which they have recently conducted in order to see (a) if a link exists between the problems encountered around the time of the climacteric and a woman's earlier menstrual experience, and (b) if social factors affect the climacteric experience.

The study was conducted in an urban community in Norway. It involved 200 women who were randomly selected, but who were aged between 45 and 55. The data were gathered by means of a postal questionnaire. Six symptom groups emerging from factor analysis were investigated; these were mood liability, vague somatic complaints, vasomotor problems, 'nervousness', urinary problems, and shortness of breath and palpitations. Of these, only vasomotor problems (hot flushes and profuse sweating) can really be regarded as being related to the climacteric. It was interesting to see, however, that the occurrence of problems *per se*, rather than menopausal status, determined whether a woman described herself as being 'climacteric' or not.

Table 1   Specific correlations between earlier menstrual experience and problems encountered in middle-age, and their common denominators

Patterns emerging from the factor analysis	Earlier menstrual experience	Problems encountered in middle-age	Common denominator
1*	Feeling depressed	Mood lability	Depression
2*	Nausea	Vague somatic problems	Somatization
3	—	Vasomotor problems	(Peri-menopausal status)
4*	Pain	'Nervousness'	Tension
5	Light bleedings	Urinary problems	Genital reactions
6	Irregular menstrual pattern	Shortness of breath, palpitations	Disturbed body rhythm

*Statistical significance, $p < 0.05$

The non-climacteric related problems were linked to the women's earlier menstrual experiences, but vasomotor problems were not (Table 1). Mood lability in middle-age was most frequently found in women who earlier in life had been troubled by feelings of depression around the time of menstruation. Vague somatic problems were linked to a history of nausea at menstruation, and 'nervousness' often occurred in women who usually experienced pain at the time of menstruation. Additionally, but not significant statistically, there was a tendency for urinary problems in middle-age to occur in women who had experienced light menstrual bleedings, and for shortness of breath and palpitations to occur in those who had experienced an irregular menstrual pattern. Intercorrelations between the different menstrual experiences were low and not statistically significant.

Only a few social background variables were shown to correlate with climacteric symptom patterns. One finding was that women who have a good social network, i.e., who have friends, particularly women friends, to whom they can talk, tend not to suffer climacteric problems of a psychological nature: mood lability, vague somatic symptoms, and 'nervousness'. The having of a personal income, but not socio-economic status, was a main determinant where vasomotor complaints were concerned; women with some income of their own tended to be less troubled by such complaints.

It seems therefore that, at least to some extent, certain aspects of women's menstrual experience can be used as pre-climacteric indicators of the likely experience of women around the time of the menopause. In view of the findings of this study it is suggested that future longitudinal studies of the development of climacteric symptoms include the registration of menstrual experience.

The paper of *Lax* dealt with the predictability, from the psycho-analytical point of view, of the woman's reaction to the climacteric being a depressive one. She quoted Benedek (1950) who said that the climacteric represents a progressive psychological adaptation to a regressive biological process. She also quoted Deutsch (1945) who pointed out that almost all women go through a phase of depression around the time of the climacteric, during which the biologic state of averse is over-emphasized. She mentioned too the findings of Severne (1979).

Lax then drew attention to the psycho-ethological reactions of women to the climacteric, in which phase-specific physiological changes become evident. These changes are expressed in the woman's self-image, in her sense of body integrity and body function, and in her life tasks and 'ego interests'. The effects of these changes are further expressed in:

(1) Restlessness, often associated with a decreased ability to concentrate
(2) Insomnia
(3) Uncontrollable vasomotor discharges, i.e., hot flushes, profuse sweating, palpitations and other cardiac discomforts.

These changes in the psycho-physical equilibrium may well evoke the risk of regressive threats.

Lax feels these problems to be accentuated in today's youth-oriented ethos in which ageing in itself evokes a sense of shame and is a process to be hidden away. She links this with experience of narcissistic loss and with infantile fears of loss of control. Such a feeling can cause increased anxiety, which, in turn, can lead to severe disturbance in sleep patterns, and a sense of fatigue, and may well contribute to generalized irritability.

The profound sense of loss and increased narcissistic vulnerability due to the ending of procreativity can be accentuated in our culture by the fact that men do not experience an ending to their procreativity. The confrontation of this biologically determined fact can reactivate many unsolved infantile emotional problems which are rooted in the oedipal phase of life.

An escape into (pathological) health is a defensive coping mechanism in the peri-menopause (Musaph, 1979). The media, the cosmetics industry, and plastic surgery, at least in the United States, help women to accept pathological health as a coping mechanism.

Bibring (1953) and Zetzel (1970) considered depression to be an integral part of psychic life, an opinion shared by *Lax*. The experience of depression is a prerequisite for optimal maturation and must be regarded as a phase-specific effect. *Lax* feels that when the 'mourning process' over lost procreation function is accompanied by a 'working through' which results in the development of greater self-tolerance and self-acceptance, object relations become enriched. Moreover, mourning, when successful, leads to an adaptive and creative restructuring of some aspects of one's wishful self-image.

Maoz, the final speaker in this section of the workshop, was not able to give any actual data, his study with *Walfish* and *Antonovsky* at the Ben Gurion University in Israel not yet being finished, but he did tell us of the thinking behind his study.

The premise is that a mid-life disturbance in the bio-psycho-social equilibrium in the life of the family unit, especially in the marital relationship, may be, if not a cause, certainly an aggravating factor in the occurrence of climacteric problems, and the real reason for help-seeking behaviour. This study, which involves 50 married parous couples, investigates independent variables such as mutual support, sexual relations, change in social rôles, and perception of menopause. The study has been carefully planned, and one looks forward with interest to learning of its findings.

INFLUENCE OF HORMONES

De Lignières has investigated the effects of exogenous oestradiol and progesterone on the mood of post-menopausal women. It has been known for some time that these two steroids have an influence on some enzymatic and electric activities of the central nervous system in primates, but their clinical effects on mood and behaviour in women are generally uncertain. There are several reasons for this.

(1) The accumulation of data from different studies is difficult, because there is not sufficient similarity in the meanings of the terms used to describe clinical problems.

(2) Few reports give precise correlations between the clinical and the endocrinological findings in individual women.

(3) The therapeutic regimens used in studies tend to be standardized, with the same daily dose being given to all patients, irrespective of their individual requirements. As a result, unpleasant symptoms due to an insufficient daily dose being given to one patient are mixed with those resulting from what is an excessive dose for another patient. This gives a completely false report on the effectiveness of the drug.

In *de Lignière*'s experience, moderate depressive symptoms, such as pessimism, fatigue, sleep disturbance, and loss of energy are often correlated in post-menopausal women with a decrease in plasma levels of oestradiol and/or of Δ4 androstenedione.

When oestradiol is given (percutaneously in *de Lignière*'s studies) the plasma oestradiol levels rise, and beneficial effects occur. When the rise is excessive, however, and levels of more than 150 pg/ml are reached, the exogenous oestradiol induces unpleasant side effects, such as pessimism, irritability, aggressiveness, and restlessness. These complaints often occur concomitantly with breast and abdominal swellings, similar to those seen in the pre-menstrual syndrome. The ideal dosages of oestradiol appear to be those which lead to plasma oestradiol levels of between 50 and 150 pg/ml.

De Lignière has also found that natural progesterone, the micronized form designed for oral use, can have a beneficial effect on mood problems when these occur in conjunction with a high level of plasma oestradiol and a low level of plasma progesterone. Here too a moderate elevation is usually all that is needed. The progesterone then has a pleasant 'tranquillizing' effect, which women describe variously as making them feel more peaceful, more self-confident, less irritable, and better able to sleep. Too high a dose, resulting in plasma levels in excess of 40 ng/ml, invariably has too strong a soporific effect.

It is clear from these observations that the administration of natural steroid preparations can indeed have a beneficial effect on the mood of post-menopausal women. It is equally clear, however, that one must carefully adapt the dose to the pharmacokinetic pattern of the individual patient, for adverse effects quickly occur when too high a dose is given.

Dennerstein spoke on female sexuality, middle-age, the menopause, and on the rôle and influence of hormones. In her opinion hormonal changes can indeed affect sexual behaviour, at least in women with stable relationships. It is important for the clinician to be aware of this when planning hormone therapy for post-menopausal women. A deficiency of oestrogen may not necessarily be the cause of sexual problems in mid-life but may provide a biological vulnerability which for women with a somewhat tenuous sexual adjustment may be enough to tip the balance from 'just coping' to sexual dysfunction. Once sexual dysfunction exists it is unlikely that oestrogen therapy alone will produce a sufficient change in behaviour because of the profound effects of social learning and of the performance anxieties which will have developed.

All women presenting with sexual problems in middle-age should receive careful assessment, an assessment aimed at delineating the problem, the level of psycho-sexual development of the woman, her inter-personal relationships, other psycho-social stresses and her attitudes to middle-age and the menopause, any psychiatric or orgasmic contribut-ing factors, including hormonal status, and thus establishing the likely aetiology of the problem.

An integrated approach to management is needed, aimed at reducing contributory hormonal, psychological and social stress, and promoting a positive adaptation to this developmental phase. Often some individual sessions with the woman are helpful in achieving this prior to commenc-ing couple therapy in which psychotherapeutic techniques are combined with structured behavioural tasks.

It has become apparent that hormones do play a modulating rôle in female human sexual behaviour. Knowledge of these effects may help the physician provide an optimal hormonal background prior to com-mencing an integrated approach to the complex problems of mid-life sexual disorders.

CONCLUSION

It became clear, not only from this workshop, but also from others which took place during this congress, that the peri-menopause syndrome is best tackled with a multi-disciplinary approach. The aetiology of the syndrome is complex. The attitude and behaviour of the male partner and of other members of the family can have great influence on the psychopathology of the woman. Problems encountered in mid-life sometimes have their origin in puberty and adolescence, unresolved problems being reactivated by the climacteric and its concurrent 'empty nest' syndrome. Such problems often affect marital relationships. Complaints such as dyspareunia, erectile difficulties, vaginal soreness, and loss of libido are easily triggered by emotional difficulties. Medical treatment in the form of hormone therapy is often helpful to women in the peri-menopause, particularly when it is combined with psychotherapy. An integrated approach to the management of the perimenopausal woman, whereby a multi-disciplinary team is available to help the entire family, is clearly to be advocated.

References

Benedek, T. (1950). Climacterium: A developmental phase. *Psychoanal. Q.*, **19**, 1

Bibring, E. (1953). The mechanisms of depression. In Greenacre, P. (ed.) *Affective Disorders*, pp. 13–48. (New York: International Universities Press)

Deutsch, H. (1945). *Psychology of Women*, Vol. 2. (New York: Grune and Stratton)

Flint, M. (1975). The menopause: reward or punishment? *Psychosomatics*, **16**, 161

Haspels, A. A. and Musaph, H. (eds.) (1979). *Psychosomatics in Peri-menopause* (Lancaster: MTP)

van Keep, P. A. and Gregory, A. (1977). Sexual relations in the ageing female. In Money, J. and Musaph, H. (eds.) *Handbook of Sexology*, Chap. 62. (Amsterdam, London, New York: Excerpta Medica)

King, P. (1980). The life cycle as indicated by the nature of the transference in the psychoanalysis of the middle-aged and elderly. *Int. J. Psycho. Anal.*, **61**, 153

Lauritzen, C. and Müller, P. (1977). Pathology and involution of the genitals in the ageing female. In Money, J. and Musaph, H.(eds.) *Handbook of Sexology*, Chap. 63. (Amsterdam, London, New York: Excerpta Medica)

Maoz, B., Antonovsky, A., Apter, A., Datan, N., Hochberg, J. and Salomon, Y. (1978). The effects of outside work on the menopausal woman. *Maturitas*, **1**, 43

Musaph, H. (1977). Skin, touch and sex. In Money, J. and Musaph, H. (eds.) *Handbook of Sexology*, Chap. 94. (Amsterdam, London, New York: Excerpta Medica)

Musaph, H. (1979). The trigger function of the menopause. In Haspels, A. A. and Musaph, H. (eds.) *Psychosomatics in Peri-menopause*, Chap. 6. (Lancaster: MTP)

Musaph, H. and Haspels, A. A. (eds.) (1977). *Dyspareunia. Aspects of Painful Coitus.* (Utrecht: Bohn, Scheltema and Holkema)

Severne, L. (1979). Psycho-social aspects of the menopause. In Haspels, A. A. and Musaph, H. (eds.) *Psychosomatics in Peri-menopause*, Chap. 7. (Lancaster: MTP)

Zetzel, E. (1970). *The Capacity for Emotional Growth.* (New York: International Universities Press)

Workshop 6

The breast

Moderator: **J. McQueen** (UK)

Speakers: **R. D. Bulbrook** (UK)
J. G. van Dijk (The Netherlands)
R. B. Greenblatt (USA)
R. Sitruk-Ware (France)
M. P. Vessey (UK)

INTRODUCTION

There are various reasons why a consideration of the breast by doctors who are caring for women in the middle years is important. The great psychological importance to the woman herself is one factor. As with the endometrium, it is a site of origin of oestrogen dependent cancer, but, whereas study of the endometrium is made relatively simple by ease of access, the exact state of a breast is, as yet, quite unable to be determined without mastectomy. The relationship between hormonal therapy and breast cancer can, therefore, only be determined by very large epidemiological studies. Benign breast disease can cause great distress to a woman, either symptomatically or because of the need for surgery to exclude malignancy. It also is a predisposing factor to breast cancer. These are the aspects which were considered in this workshop, and, as was feared, more questions were asked than could be answered.

THE PSYCHOLOGICAL IMPORTANCE OF THE BREASTS
(Presented by J. G. van Dijk)

Van Dijk gave her personal views of the psychological importance of the breasts:

(a) They are a sign of *femininity*. The timing of the development of the breasts at puberty is important for a harmonious integration of body growth and psychosexual development. Appearance too early or too late may cause frustrations that influence the personal value of the organs for a very long time.

(b) The breasts also contribute to *security and oral satisfaction*. Their physiological function is to feed the child who, in addition to nutrition, derives security from the warm skin and, possibly, even the maternal heartbeat. This may be important for the child's ability to love and enjoy its own body and sensuality. The mother also derives much from this relationship with the baby.

(c) The breasts are also, of course, deeply involved in a woman's *sexuality*, and give her a degree of power over men.

PROGESTERONE AND BENIGN BREAST DISEASE
(Presented by R. Sitruk-Ware)

Experimental fibrocystic disease of the breast can be caused in castrated mice by administering oestrogen. If progesterone is also given, a complete and proper breast development occurs. In benign breast diseases Sitruk-Ware *et al.* (1979) have suggested, as a result of hormonal investigation of 184 patients, that a progesterone insufficiency is the main pathological component. They measured oestradiol and progesterone levels during the luteal phase of patients suffering from benign breast disease who were ovulating, as determined by a biphasic temperature chart. These were compared with levels in normal controls. The progesterone levels were significantly lower in the patients while the oestradiol levels were normal or raised. The ratio of plasma progesterone to oestradiol levels was very significantly lower in the affected patients.

There is very little information about hormone receptors in benign breast lesions as much of the breast structure is not hormone dependent. Martin *et al.* (1978) have studied 84 fibroadenomas removed surgically, and found that there is a high level of oestradiol receptors when epithelial cell density was predominant compared with the degree of fibrosis.

These tumours were generally found in young women (mean age 25) and had recently appeared. The level of oestradiol receptors diminished the longer the period of evolution of the tumour and the greater the fibrosis in relation to epithelial cells. Progesterone receptors were present only in the most cellular tumours. In these cellular tumours changes in the menstrual cycle in the distribution of cytoplasmic and nuclear oestradiol and progesterone receptors are very similar to those noticed in human endometrium. There is a progressive increase in cytoplasmic and nuclear oestrogen receptors during the follicular phase, and a striking decrease in the luteal phase reflecting the anti-oestrogenic activity of progesterone. Progesterone receptors reach a high level at the end of the follicular phase due to oestrogenic stimulation, and thereafter the effect of progesterone is to cause an overall decrease in progesterone receptors, but with a relative increase in the proportion in the nucleus. In fibroadenomas there is a rise in cytoplasmic progesterone receptors, possibly reflecting the inadequate luteal phase in these patients. With progestogen treatment there is a marked translocation into the nucleus.

Since 1972, 880 women with benign mastopathy have been treated with topical applications of percutaneous progesterone alone and associated with oral progestogens. There were three groups of patients:

(1) those suffering from mastodynia alone
(2) those with increased nodularity of both breasts with predominant areas in the upper outer quadrants of both breasts
(3) those with fibroadenomas, cysts and fibrocystic disease.

They were assessed clinically, mammographically, and by thermography. Locally applied gel containing 50 mg progesterone/day completely relieved mastodynia in 73.8% of patients. There was a clinical improvement in cases of increased nodularity, whereas it was almost ineffective in the third group. The addition of oral progestogens did, however, produce a significant improvement.

Mammographic improvement was less significant as changes in breast oedema are not easily detected by this method. Intralobular sclerosis is unchanged by hormonal therapy.

Thermography demonstrates very well the effect of the treatment. In normal breasts there is a progressive rise in temperature of 1° to 2°C from the beginning to the end of the menstrual cycle as the vascularity of the breasts increases. In patients with mastodynia the mammary temperature is higher even at the beginning of the cycle with vascular patterns characterized by large vessels from the post-menstrual period onwards. Topical progesterone caused a normalization of the vascular pictures in 78% of those with mastodynia alone, in 80% of those with increased nodularity, and in 75% of cases of fibrocystic disease. Best results were obtained in women under 40 years of age, in whom mastodynia had recently appeared, and where there was no associated mass.

In post-menopausal women treated with oestradiol, the occurrence of mastodynia was related to the high plasma levels of oestradiol, and could be relieved by progestogen administration for 10 days each month.

These workers believe that mastodynia is the very first effect of excessive oestrogen action in the breast, and is the first symptom of benign breast disease. Progesterone or progestogen treatment is most likely to succeed at an early stage of the process when progesterone receptors are present.

DANAZOL IN THE MANAGEMENT OF MASTOPATHIES
(Presented by R. B. Greenblatt)

Greenblatt described how, in treating women for endometriosis with danazol, the fortuitous observation was made that the symptoms of fibrocystic disease of the breast were attenuated. This use of danazol has subsequently been studied. It is given in doses of 100, 200 and 400 mg/day, the dose depending on the severity of the disease. Side effects are relatively trivial, dose-dependent, and always reversible. There were no cases of thromboembolism and no vascular accidents. Treatment was given for three to six months. Ovulatory peaks of luteinizing hormone production were totally inhibited at a dose of 200 mg/day, but ovulation did occur on 100 mg/day. Prolactin levels fell precipitously in thirty to sixty days. Xeromammography was performed to exclude breast carcinoma.

The effect of the treatment was to induce a substantial reduction in nodularity of the breasts, a high proportion having complete elimination of nodules. Mastodynia was almost always greatly reduced. Danazol was particularly effective in the younger age group. Following cessation of treatment there was a return of some pain or tenderness in about one third of the patients, but the fact that nodularity disappeared, or was considerably reduced, removed much of their anxiety and fear. Thermographically there was return to a normal temperature pattern, and on xeromammography there was a reduction in density and the fibrous component of the fibrocystic disease. There was also an overall reduction in breast size.

The effect of this treatment is to spare many women unnecessary breast biopsies, and in those where nodules persist after treatment, biopsy can be more accurately directed to a localized part of the breast. It is important, however, that the possibility of breast cancer is always considered.

The mode of action of danazol therapy in benign breast disease remains uncertain. It seems to have a direct anti-oestrogenic effect on the breast tissue, and an indirect action by reducing the level of circulating steroid hormones by inhibition of pituitary hormone production and the steroidogenic process in the ovary.

THE RELATIONSHIP BETWEEN CHANGES OF PROLACTIN SECRETION AT THE MENOPAUSE AND BREAST CANCER (Presented by R. D. Bulbrook)

The menopause is an important factor in the aetiology of breast cancer. An early menopause decreases the risk while a late menopause increases it. In women whose ovaries are removed below the age of 40 the occurrence of breast cancer is one quarter of that expected (Feinlieb 1968).

The incidence of breast cancer increases steadily up to the menopause, then there is a slowing down of the rate for about five years, and then a resumed increase at a lower rate than in the pre-menopausal years.

The most likely explanation is the obvious one – that the menopause affects the incidence of breast cancer by the diminution of oestrogen stimulus. There is, however, a lack of formal evidence for the assumption that oestrogens are the most important hormones involved in breast carcinogenesis and promotion. Very little consideration has been given to other hormones and, in particular, it is worth looking at prolactin which is a powerful promoter of breast tumour growth in some animal models. Pearson (1969), working with induced breast tumours in the rat, showed that, following the triple operation of adrenalectomy, oophorectomy, and hypophysectomy, tumour growth regresses. Further growth can then be stimulated by prolactin but not by oestrogen.

Bulbrook and his co-workers have been measuring the prolactin levels in a large normal population in the island of Guernsey. About 4,000 women have had samples taken. There is a significant rise in prolactin values up to the menopause, at which time there is a 50% drop in level, followed by a secondary rise 20 years later.

Both oestrogen and prolactin levels, therefore, fall at the menopause. This may represent a reduction in carcinogenic dose, or a fall in the concentration of a tumour promoter. The incidence of lung cancer following cessation of smoking is very similar in pattern to that of breast cancer after the menopause. There is an initial decrease followed by a resumption in rate some years later. It may be, therefore, that prolactin may, like smoking, have its main function as a late stage promoter of tumour growth. The risk of lung cancer is related to the square of the dose of tobacco smoke multiplied by the fifth power of the length of time of exposure. If the effect of hormones on breast cancer is similar, very abnormal endocrine levels would not be necessary to increase the incidence. Levels towards the top of the normal range, and a few extra years of exposure, due perhaps to a late menopause, would cause a very marked increase. Indeed, prolactin levels at the higher end of the normal range have been found in high risk groups for cancer of the breast in the Guernsey study. These are women with a family history of breast cancer, obese multiparous women, and patients with benign disease of the breast. This is consistent with a role for prolactin in the aetiology of breast cancer. Further evidence for this comes from a prospective study of the women in Guernsey. Forty-two have developed breast cancer an average of five years after giving blood for prolactin estimation. The levels of prolactin have been compared with matched controls. There is no clear correlation between prolactin levels and breast cancer in women in the pre and peri-menopausal years, but there is in those at least five years after the menopause. In these the mean value is at or above the 70 percentile of the controls.

There is, therefore, some evidence to support the hypothesis that prolactin is involved in breast carcinogenesis, possibly as a late stage promoter. This could mean that preventive medicine may be possible quite late in reproductive life.

THE EPIDEMIOLOGY OF BREAST CANCER ASSOCIATED WITH OESTROGEN THERAPY (Presented by M. P. Vessey)

The known association between endogenous sex hormone production and breast cancer provides good reason to believe that exogenous hormone administration is likely to be related, in one way or another, to the risk of breast cancer. Epidemiological data are available concerning the effect of hormonal administration in three situations:

(1) during pregnancy

(2) as oral contraception

(3) as hormonal replacement therapy.

It must, however, be remembered when studying these data that there have, in many cases, been changes in preparations and that the possible carcinogenic effects of treatment may relate principally to treatment regimes that have been discontinued. Also the time in life of exposure to hormones such as oral contraceptive steroids may be of special significance, and there has been a marked change in the pattern of prescribing these substances over the years.

(1) Administration during pregnancy

There are three studies providing data about the risks of breast cancer in women treated with stilboestrol in pregnancy. The information available from these is inconclusive, but slightly worrying.

(2) Administration as oral contraceptives

A large number of epidemiological studies have been published concerning the relationship between oral contraceptives and benign lesions of the breast. These data are remarkably consistent in showing that the use of oral contraceptives decreases the incidence of benign disease of the breast, and that this effect is most pronounced in long-term users. In addition, there is evidence that the effect is attributable to the progestogen component of the pill, and that the benefit soon wears off after discontinuation.

In view of the known positive association between chronic cystic disease of the breast and breast cancer, some have inferred that combined oral contraceptives are likely to protect from breast cancer. However, Livolsi *et al.* (1978) after careful histological review of over two hundred biopsy specimens, have suggested that the pill only protects against the forms of chronic cystic disease in which epithelial atypia is minimal or absent, and which are unlikely to be associated with an increased risk of malignancy.

Published epidemiological studies of the relationship between oral contraceptives and breast cancer are of three main types. Those comparing trends in pill usage and breast cancer incidence have not given any cause for concern. Case control studies have yielded reassuring findings except that a few authors have suggested that, some women already at an increased risk of breast cancer as a result of a past history of benign breast disease, or a late first pregnancy, may have their risk heightened by taking the pill. Very large studies would be necessary to confirm or refute these suggestions. In addition, Pike *et al.* (1981) have recently suggested that prolonged use of oral contraceptives prior to the first pregnancy may increase the risk of breast cancer. *Vessey*'s own figures do not support this (Vessey *et al.* 1979). Jick *et al.* (1980a) have shown figures suggesting that women who continue to use oral contraception beyond the age of 45 have an increased risk of cancer. The third epidemiological approach is that of the large cohort studies which have not, as yet, contributed any significant amount of data to the discussion. Clearly there is a lot more information to come about the relationship between oral contraceptives and breast cancer.

(3) Administration as oestrogen replacement therapy

In contrast to work with oral contraceptives, studies up to 1976 on the association between oestrogen replacement therapy and breast cancer were of the cohort type. They were mostly not sufficiently sound epidemiologically to be interpretable. The papers of Burch (1975) and of Hoover (1976) however were important, and suggested that the risk of breast cancer might be increased by oestrogen therapy. Hoover *et al.* found that the relative risk increased with duration of follow-up, progressing to 2.0 after fifteen years. More recent cohort studies have produced negative results, but are either too small or epidemiologically fragile to contribute much to the controversy.

Sophisticated case control studies are beginning to appear in the literature, and are providing confusing results. Ross *et al.* (1980) showed an increased risk rising to a relative risk of 2.5 in women on large doses of oestrogen for several years which was only shown in women with intact ovaries. In contrast, Brinton *et al.* (1981) found the risk mostly concentrated in those with bilateral oophorectomy (relative risk 1.5). In this study the risk was found to increase with dosage of oestrogen and length of time of administration. Jick *et al.* (1980b), principally concerned with current users, found little association in hysterectomized women, but a positive association in those who had experienced a natural menopause (relative risk 3.4) and in particular in those in the age group 45–54 (relative risk 10.2). They did, however, state that they felt these findings should be considered tentative until substantiated by other studies and by detailed exploration of the way the effect varies with age and duration of dose. *Vessey* concluded that the data were confusing, but, on balance, slightly worrying. The association between breast cancer and hormone replacement therapy will be difficult to elucidate.

CONCLUSIONS

Breast pain is a symptom commonly discussed with doctors in a menopause clinic. It may be associated with, or a precursor to, structural benign disease of the breast. This, in turn, may predispose to breast cancer. Breast pain is a symptom of excessive oestrogenic stimulation of the breasts. If a woman is complaining of mastodynia, she is not suffering from oestrogen lack, and this symptom is unlikely to co-exist with hot flushes on any one day. If she is not receiving exogenous oestrogen, she is best treated with progestogens. There may well be an associated menstrual disturbance that will concomitantly be rectified by this therapy. If she is receiving oestrogen therapy for menopausal symptoms, the dose is excessive or she needs progestogen supplementation.

Should women who have had a hysterectomy always have progestogens as part of their hormone replacement therapy? It was the opinion of the great majority of those present at the workshop that they should. The epidemiological evidence concerning breast cancer and oestrogen replacement therapy is worrying. It is of note that very little attention has been paid to whether progestogens are included in the treatment regime of patients in these studies. It is probable that the endometrial cancer problem has been solved by adding progestogens to therapy. Perhaps breast cancer could be prevented at the same time.

References

Brinton, L. A., Hoover, R. N., Szklo, M. and Fraumeni, J. F. Jr. (1981). Menopausal estrogen use and risk of breast cancer. *Cancer*, **47**, 2517

Burch, J. C., Byrd, B. F. and Vaughn W. K. (1975). The effects of long-term estrogen administration to women following hysterectomy. In van Keep, P. A. and Lauritzen, C. (eds.) *Estrogens in the Post-menopause*, Front. Hormone Res., 3, pp. 208–214. (Basel: Karger)

Feinleib, M. (1968). Breast cancer and artificial menopause. A cohort study. *J. Natl. Cancer Inst.*, **41**, 315

Hoover, R., Gray, L. A. Sr., Cole, P. and MacMahon, B. (1976). Menopausal estrogens and breast cancer. *N. Engl. J. Med.*, **295**, 401

Jick, H., Walker, A. M., Watkins, R. N., D'Ewart, D. C., Hunter, J. R., Danford, D. A., Madsen, S., Dinan, B. J. and Rothman, K. J. (1980a). Oral contraceptives and breast cancer. *Am. J. Epidemiol.*, **112**, 577

Jick, H., Walker, A. M., Watkins, R. N., D'Ewart, D. C., Hunter, J. R., Danford, D. A., Madsen, S., Dinan, B. J. and Rothman, K. J. (1980b). Replacement estrogens and breast cancer. *Am. J. Epidemiol.*, **112**, 586

Livolsi, V. A., Stadel, B. V., Kelsey, J. L., Holford, T. R. and White, C. (1978). Fibro-cystic disease in oral contraceptive users. A histopathological evaluation of epithelial atypia. *N. Engl. J. Med.*, **299**, 381

Martin, P., Kuttenn, F., Serment, H. and Mauvais-Jarvis, P. (1978). Studies on clinical, hormonal, and pathological correlations in breast fibroadenomas. *J. Steroid Biochem.*, **9**, 1251

Pearson, O. H., Llerena, O., Llerena, L., Molina, A. and Butler, T. (1969). Prolactin-dependant rat mammary cancer: A model for man? *Trans. Assoc. Am. Physicians*, **82**, 225

Pike, M. C., Henderson, B. E., Casagrande, J. T., Rosario, I. and Gray, G. E. (1981). Oral contraceptive use and early abortion as risk factors for breast cancer in young women. *Br. J. Cancer*, **43**, 72

Ross, R. K., Paganini-Hill, A., Gerkins, V. R., Mack, T. M. Pfeffer, R., Arthur, M. and Henderson, B. E. (1980). A case-control study of menopausal estrogen therapy and breast cancer. *J. Am. Med. Assoc.*, **243**, 1635

Sitruk-Ware, R., Sterkers, N. and Mauvais-Jarvis, P. (1979). Benign breast diseases. Part. 1. Hormonal investigations. *Obstet. Gynecol.*, **53**, 457

Vessey, M. P., Doll, R., Jones, K., McPherson, K. and Yeates, D. (1979). An epidemio-logical study of oral contraceptives and breast cancer. *Br. Med. J.*, i, 1757

Workshop 7

Neuroendocrine changes in the peri-menopause

Moderators: **U. J. Gaspard** (Belgium)
             P. Franchimont (Belgium)

Speakers: **P. Aschheim** (France)
             S. Ballinger (Australia)
             J. P. Bourguignon (Belgium)
             D. A. Davey (South Africa)
             A. Demoulin (Belgium)
             P. Franchimont (Belgium)
             U. J. Gaspard (Belgium)
             H. S. Jacobs (UK)
             G. Langer (Austria)
             P. Linkowski (Belgium)
             J. C. Stevenson (UK)

THE HYPOTHALAMIC-PITUITARY-OVARIAN AXIS AT THE MENOPAUSE

In the human species follicular depletion of the ovaries and exhaustion of their gametogenic and endocrine functions are somewhat precocious events. They result in irregular, frequently anovulatory, cycles and finally in menopausal amenorrhoea. Within two years after the menopause the ovaries secrete only insignificant quantities of oestrogens but still substantial amounts of androgens. Oestrone becomes the major circulating post-menopausal oestrogen and this arises almost entirely from the peripheral conversion of androstenedione. This latter hormone originates mainly from the adrenals and to a lesser extent from the ovaries. The decrease in circulating oestrogens after the menopause is attended by a dramatic elevation in blood levels of FSH and LH reflecting an increased production of both these gonadotrophins in the absence of a negative feed-back system.

Following bilateral oophorectomy, plasma oestradiol falls rapidly to one-tenth, plasma oestrone to one-half, and total urinary oestrogens to one-fifteenth of the pre-operative levels, and all remain low (*Davey*). Concurrently, plasma androstenedione levels fall to one-half of antecedent concentrations, but plasma testosterone remains unchanged. Thus, it is evident that oophorectomized women are oestrogen deficient. No compensatory changes have been seen during an 18 months period of observation. The FSH levels rise progressively in the first six months after oophorectomy, reaching a maximum of four times or more the pre-operative level, and LH similarly rises, to double or more.

This comparatively greater increase in FSH over LH results in FSH:LH ratios of >1.

The endocrine profile depicted after oophorectomy is rather similar to the hormonal status of post-menopausal women. However, castration after the menopause results in an additional increase in gonadotrophin concentrations. This illustrates the persistence of a negative feed-back mechanism possibly due to androstenedione and testosterone of ovarian origin, or their peripheral metabolites. On the other hand, in immediately pre-menopausal women, LH, oestradiol and progesterone are within the normal range during the menstrual cycle, but the values of FSH may be increased (Sherman *et al.*, 1976). Therefore, the disturbance in the regulation of FSH secretion in the peri-menopausal phase cannot be explained only in terms of steroid modifications.

A protein hormone called inhibin, which originates in the gonads and regulates FSH secretion, has recently been described by several groups (for a review see Franchimont *et al.*, 1979). Inhibin is synthesized by Sertoli cells in the male and by granulosa cells in the female, and can be found in ovarian extracts, follicular, and peritoneal fluid (but only after rupture of the follicle). Injected immediately after castration in the rat, inhibin prevents the FSH rise by a direct action at the pituitary level. Inhibin preparations also prevent synthesis and release of FSH by rat pituitary cells in culture under basal conditions and in the presence of LHRH.

In a preliminary experiment by *Demoulin et al.*, ovaries were surgically removed from one pre-menopausal and from one post-menopausal woman. After absorption of the steroids and protein estimation, the ovarian extracts were biologically tested for their content of inhibin, which was estimated to be 3863 mU/mg protein in the pre-menopausal but only 357 mU/mg protein in the post-menopausal woman (Figure 1).

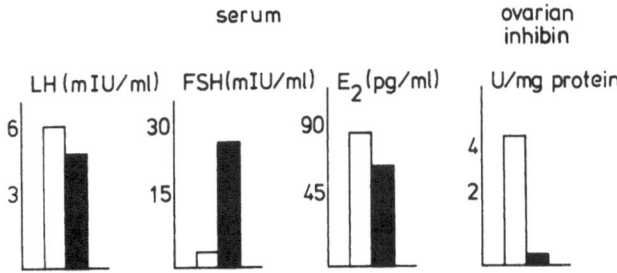

Figure 1 Serum levels of LH, FSH, and oestradiol (E_2) and the ovarian content of inhibin expressed in units/mg protein (international standard, Hudson *et al.*, 1979), in an eumenorrhoeic pre-menopausal woman aged 42 years (open bars) and in an oligomenorrhoeic climacteric woman aged 48 years (closed bars) presenting with elevated serum levels of FSH. (*Demoulin et al.*)

Although restricted to only two observations, this preliminary study may help to explain the preferential increase in FSH levels observed during the peri-menopausal phase.

Besides gonadal steroids and inhibin, which apparently play an important role in the control of gonadotrophin secretion through their feed-back actions, hypothalamic secretion of LHRH has also to be considered, as its pulsatile release, mainly from the medial basal hypothalamus in primates, is now thought to be the permissive prerequisite for pituitary gonadotrophic function (for a review see Knobil, 1980).

In menopausal or castrated humans, as well as in eugonadal subjects, LH and FSH concentrations in blood are pulsatile, with circhoral variation intervals. These pulsatile discharges of gonadotrophins seem to follow synchronous pulsatile discharges of LHRH.

As LHRH is released in minute amounts in the portal blood of the pituitary stalk and rapidly submitted to degradation and disappearance from peripheral blood, its assay in circulating blood is difficult, and, in fact, of limited value. Since LHRH has been found to be excreted in urine, it was tempting to further characterize the properties of urinary immunoreactive LHRH, to apply its assay to females in normal and in pathologic conditions at different ages, and to investigate its correlation with gonadotrophins excreted in urine. In well-defined experimental conditions, Bourguignon *et al.* (1979) have described an assay of LHRH and its 2–10 nonapeptide fragment in urine. A clear-cut increase in urinary LHRH excretion was observed in post-menopausal women compared to prepubertal girls and to eugonadal women during the follicular and luteal phases (Figure 2). However, no correlation could be

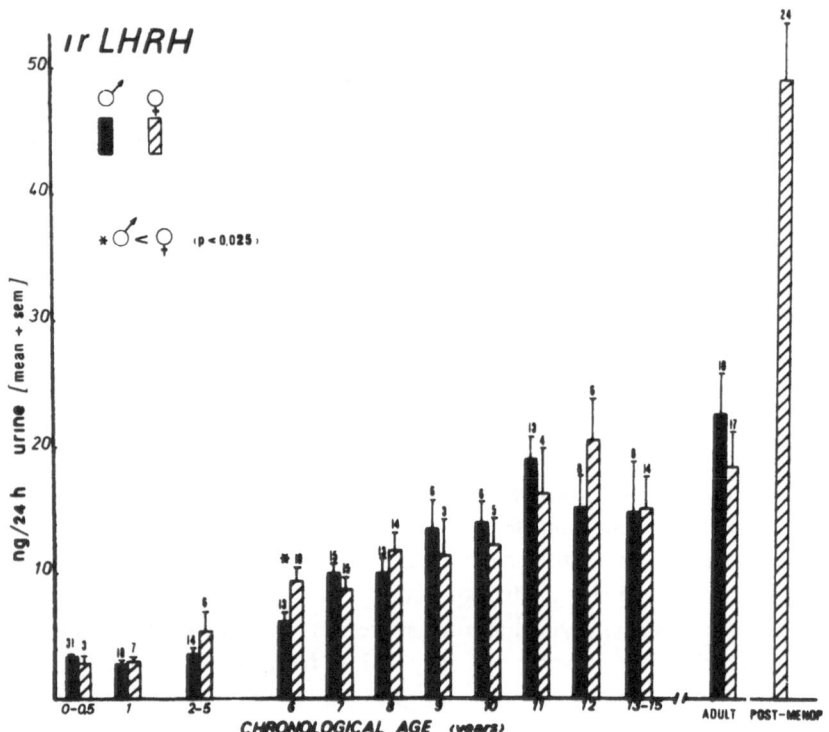

Figure 2   Mean excretion of IR-LHRH (+ SEM) in urine in different age groups of males and females. The group less than 6 months old has no neonates before two weeks of age. (From Bourguigon *et al.*, 1979. Reproduced with permission)

seen between the levels of urinary IR-LHRH and gonadotrophins. Nevertheless the finding of increased IR-LHRH in urine of post-menopausal women suggests the existence of a negative feed-back effect of gonadal steroids at the hypothalamic level. In spite of these observations, many questions remain unanswered: What is the exact pulsatile pattern of LHRH at the menopause and its amplitude? Why should elevated endogenous LHRH secretion by the hypothalamus not induce a 'down regulation' at the level of the pituitary? To what extent are sex steroids, neurotransmitters, and possibly inhibin involved in the regulation of LHRH secretion in the post-menopause? etc.

A detailed study of the endocrine and neuroendocrine mechanisms involved in the menopausal process necessarily involves the use of animal models. Low cost, ready availability, and a short life-span between birth, cessation of ovarian function, and death are interesting features of animal models. Nevertheless, ovarian exhaustion in the human female is a precocious ageing process and the majority of women experience a post-menopausal phase lasting one-third or more of lives. By comparison, female monkeys, certain strains of mice ($C_{57}B_1$), and rats experience an anoestrus period of only 10–15% of their lifetime. Hypothalamic and pituitary ageing processes seem to be more deeply involved in these animal species than in women (Peng and Huang, 1972) and caution regarding the selection of a suitable animal model for the human menopause is mandatory. Attention has recently focused on the mouse of the CBA strain which lives for an average of some 530 days and displays virtually complete depletion of ovarian oocytes by 300–400 days. Data pointing to an intrinsic ovarian ageing in this strain have recently been obtained (*Aschheim*). From 12 months on, FSH and LH levels are much higher in these anoestrous mice than at 4 months (cyclic mice), but comparable to the gonadotrophin levels observed in castrated 4 month-old mice. The very few females with normal FSH concentrations after 12 months of age retain growing follicles in their ovaries. An important age-related weight regression of the ovaries is recorded from 12 months onwards, simultaneously with exhaustion of the secretory activity of the steroidogenic cells. These observations suggest that the CBA mouse may be the best animal model available at present for the study of human ovarian ageing process.

NEUROENDOCRINE CHANGES UNDERLYING CLIMACTERIC FLUSHING

Neurocirculatory dysregulation frequently occurs around the time of the menopause resulting in hot flushes and profuse perspiration. It has been reported that 65–75% of women are affected by this, and that in some 25–50% of women these hot flushes are experienced for five years or even longer (Benedek-Jaszmann, 1976). According to Meldrum *et al.* (1979), the physiological events accompanying a hot flush are as follows: early central recognition preceding the hot flush sometimes causing the woman to wake if she is asleep, development of the hot flush with lowering of tympanic (central) temperature, increase in peripheral cutaneous conduction and temperature for up to 20–40 min, and increase in heart rate and hand blood flow (it must be remembered that a rich complex of α-adrenergic terminals is present in the hands). Our present understanding of the mechanism underlying climacteric flushing is limited. Hot flushes occur commonly after the menopause and ovariectomy, and, although less frequently, in hypogonadal and agonadal subjects (including males), i.e., in cases of low circulating sex steroids (particularly oestrogens) accompanied or not by elevated concentrations of gonadotrophins. Oestrogen treatment abolishes climacteric flushing. However, numerous cases of hyperprolactinaemia, or anorexia nervosa presenting with severe hypooestrogenism exhibit no episodes of flushing. Blood sampling coupled with early recognition of the discharge of an impending hot flush, and increasing finger temperature, has shown that increased LH is an early and regular event accompanying the hot flush, whereas it is not possible to relate attacks of flushing to particular concentrations of conjugated or unconjugated ('free') oestradiol or oestrone in blood. In recent experiments *Jacobs* and his group were not able to demonstrate any significant variations in the circulating levels of FSH, prolactin, or oestrogens during the initiation period of hot flushes. They confirmed that a significant increase in LH (more than 25% over basal levels) can be observed with each flush and that a simultaneous drop in circulating norepinephrine is sometimes recorded (Lightman *et al.*, 1981).

There is some evidence that alcohol and enkephalin and its analogues are capable of inducing flushing and of altering LH secretion, implying that LH secretion could be at least partially under the control of endogenous opiate receptor stimulation. Conversely, Genazzani has recently reported an increase in blood levels of β-endorphin and opioids after the onset of hot flushes (personal communication). A new finding of *Jacobs et al.* is that infusion of naloxone (an opiate antagonist) in climacteric women inhibits the occurrence of flushing and markedly depresses LH pulsatility (correlation coefficient $r = 0.85$) (Figure 3). LH pulsatility was unchanged under naloxone infusion in only one instance, and in that subject flushing episodes were also unaltered. However, selective inhibition of LH release can be effected at the level of the pituitary (but not of the hypothalamus) by the down regulation mechanism induced by the administration of superactive analogues of LHRH. In that case, effective suppression of LH pulsatile discharges was obtained, but it was

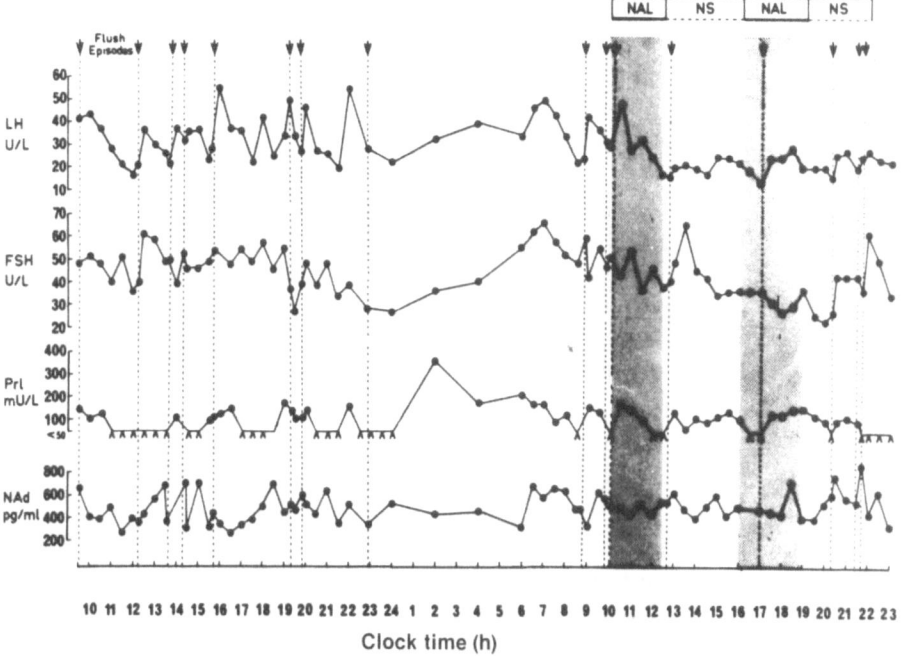

Figure 3 Plasma LH, FSH, prolactin (Prl) and noradrenaline (NAd) concentrations measured at 30 minute intervals in one subject. The times of perception of a flush are indicated by the vertical arrows. Naloxone (NAL) and saline (NS) were infused on the second day of observation. (Lightman *et al.*)

not attended by any decrease in climacteric flushing, suggesting that no causal relation exists between pituitary gonadotrophin secretion and the generation of hot flushes. In confirmation of this observation Judd (1981) recently reported that in two patients in whom craniopharyngioma was surgically removed in association with hypophysectomy, characteristic hot flushes developed in spite of the absence of LH discharges. So hot flushes and LH discharges in some way respond to a common (opiate?) triggering mechanism without sharing a causal relationship. Oestrogens or their metabolites may alter hypothalamic control of LH release and temperature regulation by increasing the turnover rate of cerebral catecholamines, by exerting a central antidopaminergic action, or, possibly, by inhibiting opiate-receptor interactions (*Jacobs et al.*). The potentially active metabolite is not a catecholoestrogen – or, at least, it is not 2-OH oestradiol – since infusion of this steroid into post-menopausal women does not succeed in altering LH release or flushing. The problem requires further work, particularly since there is a fairly large group of women presenting with this distressing symptom, for whom, for medical reasons, treatment with oestrogens is contra-indicated.

ROLE OF OESTROGENS IN CALCITONIN AND PARATHYROID HORMONE SECRETION

It is well-recognized that loss of ovarian function leads to loss of bone in women. Furthermore, this bone loss can be arrested or even reversed by oestrogen therapy. The mechanism of this action of oestrogen is not clear, as oestrogen has not been shown to act directly on bone. Circulating calcitonin levels are low and display a circadian rhythm with a peak concentration at twelve noon and a nadir at midnight. Mean levels of immunoreactive calcitonin in eugonadal women are about 20 pg/ml (sometimes undetectable), whereas concentrations in adult men are more than twice that level. Interestingly, women taking oral contraceptive agents have calcitonin levels in the male range (*Stevenson*). Calcitonin concentrations decline with ageing in both sexes, but the occurrence of menopause or castration accelerates this phenomenon and the lack of oestrogens is associated with calcitonin deficiency. Conversely, endogenous oestrogens (in eugonadal and pregnant women) or exogenous oestrogens increase calcitonin levels. In contradistinction to calcitonin levels, parathormone concentrations are only minimally influenced by endogenous or exogenous oestrogens and the post-menopausal drop in circulating parathormone is minimal. Thus, women are normally relatively deficient in calcitonin compared to men, and since calcitonin protects against bone resorption directed by dihydroxycholecalciferol and parathormone, the female skeleton already in physiological conditions is more sensitive to the actions of bone-resorbing hormones.

Loss of oestrogens at the climacteric accelerates the natural decline of calcitonin secretion that occurs with age. Thus, the post-menopausal woman has the most exaggerated calcitonin deficiency which leads to a relative increase in bone resorption, even though actual levels of bone-resorbing hormones are not increased. In women with precocious meno-pause, where oestrogen deprivation occurs, calcitonin deficiency is also clearly demonstrable, though not age-related in that case (*Stevenson*). The overall result of calcitonin deficiency is loss of bone. Oestrogen appears to act favourably on bone, at least in part, via calcitonin. Thus, the combination of oestrogen and calcitonin deficiency appears to be a most important factor in the pathogenesis of post-menopausal bone loss.

NEUROENDOCRINE CHANGES IN DEPRESSED PRE- AND POST-MENOPAUSAL WOMEN

Depression is a frequently presenting illness in the peri-menopause. Disturbances in mood, appetite, sleep, sexual drive and circadian rhythmicity are symptoms usually found in association with depression, but they can also occur as a result of hypothalamic dysfunction. Moreover, neurotransmitters, putatively responsible for the pathogenesis of depression, are also implicated in the secretory functions of the hypothalamo-pituitary axis and could potentially reflect in the hormonal secretory dynamics they modulate. These are the two main reasons to postulate that major depressive illnesses are associated with disorders of the neuroendocrine function, and to support neuroendocrine investigations in depressive syndromes (*Linkowski*).

Langer and *Linkowski* agree that in unipolar depressive post-menopausal women, TSH response to TRH is significantly lower than in post-menopausal controls. The same observation has been made by *Langer* for unipolar depression in pre-menopausal women, in association with somewhat elevated serum thyroxine levels. In bipolar depression, TSH response to TRH is blunted during the pre-menopause but normal in the post-menopause.

Prolactin response to TRH and to an insulin tolerance test is blunted in post-menopausal depressive women. The causes of these lowered TSH and prolactin responses to TRH or insulin tests in subgroups of bipolar or unipolar depressive women before and after the menopause are incompletely understood and are probably multifactorial, possibly involving the effects of cortisol production which is often increased in depressive subjects, the severity of the mental illness, and so on. Thus, the role of abnormalities in neurotransmitter secretion and metabolism is possible but must be elucidated. The pattern of neuroendocrine parameters possibly affected by menopausal status have not yet been interpreted on the grounds of deductive reasoning based on a sufficient amount of experimental data. Furthermore, it is becoming evident that pituitary hormones are not the best parameters for assessing the metabolism of the central nervous system and that more attention should be paid to more specific neurohormones, such as endorphins, enkephalins, melatonin, substance P, etc.

The roles of oestrogens and of their metabolites have also to be taken into consideration in post-menopausal depression. Probably the strongest evidence on the mechanisms of depression to date lies in the hypothesis of a catecholamine deficit in depression. In post-menopausal depressive women an inverse relationship exists between the concentrations of urinary oestradiol, oestrone, and total oestrogens, and the severity of the depression (*Ballinger*). The same observation is also true for plasma oestrone, for oestradiol, and for total urinary catecholoestrogens. This latter observation may be of some importance as catecholoestrogens are strong competitors for catechol-*o*-methyltransferase (COMT), a major enzyme catabolizing dopamine and noradrenalin. High levels of catecholoestrogens in the brain would leave less COMT available for noradrenalin breakdown. This, theoretically, would leave more noradrenalin available in the brain and may potentiate its action (Klaiber *et al.*, 1979). Therefore additional information concerning catecholoestrogen levels and their physiologic action in post-menopausal women and depressive patients is desirable.

References

Benedek-Jaszmann, L. J. (1976). Epidemiology of the climacteric syndrome. In Campbell, S. (ed.) *The Management of the Menopause and Post-menopausal Years*, pp. 11–23. (Lancaster: MTP Press)

Bourguignon, J. P., Hoyoux, C., Reuter, A., Franchimont, P., Lewartz-Dourcy, C. and Vrindts-Gevaert, Y. (1979). Urinary excretion of immunoreactive luteinizing hormone-releasing hormone-like material and gonadotropins at different stages of life. *J. Clin. Endocrinol. Metab.*, **48**, 78

Franchimont, P., Verstraelen-Proyard, J., Hazee-Hagelstein, M. T., Renard, Ch., Demoulin, A., Bourguignon, J. P. and Hustin, J. (1979). Inhibin: From concept to reality. *Vitam. Horm.*, **37**, 243

Hudson, B., Baker, H. W. G., Eddie, L. W., Higginson, R. E., Burger, H. G., de Kretser, D. M., Dobos, M. and Lee, V. W. K. (1979). Bioassays for inhibin: a critical review. *J. Reprod. Fertil.*, suppl. 26, 17

Judd, H. L. (1982). Pathophysiology of the hot flush. In Flamigni, C. and Givens, J. R. (eds.) *The Gonadotrophins: Basic Science and Clinical Aspects in Females.* (London: Academic Press) (In press)

Klaiber, E. L., Broverman, D. M., Vogel, W. and Kobayashi, Y. (1979). Estrogen therapy for severe persistent depressions in women. *Arch. Gen. Psychiatry*, **36**, 550

Knobil, E. (1980). The neuroendocrine control of the menstrual cycle. *Recent Prog. Horm. Res.*, **36**, 53

Lightman, S. L., Jacobs, H. S., Maguire, A. K., McGarrick, G. and Jeffcoate, S. L. (1981). Climacteric flushing: clinical and endocrine response to infusion of Naloxone. *Br. J. Obstet. Gynaecol.* (In press)

Meldrum, D. R., Shamonki, I. M., Frumar, A. M., Tataryn, I. V., Chang, R. J. and Judd, H. L. (1979). Elevation in skin temperature of the finger as an objective index of postmenopausal hot flushes: Standardization of the technique. *Am. J. Obstet. Gynecol.*, **135**, 713

Peng, M. and Huang, H. (1972). Aging of hypothalamic-pituitary-ovarian function in the rat. *Fertil. Steril.*, **23**, 535

Sherman, B. M., West, J. H. and Korenman, S. G. (1976). The menopausal transition: Analysis of LH, FSH, estradiol, and progesterone concentrations during menstrual cycles of older women. *J. Clin. Endocrinol. Metab.*, **42**, 629

Workshop 8

Hysterectomy

Moderator: **E. V. van Hall** (The Netherlands)

Speakers: **P. M. G. H. Buytaert** (Belgium)
E. Cohen (Israel)
L. Dennerstein (Australia)
J. G. van Dijk (The Netherlands)
B. Ehret (West Germany)
J. Ovadia (Israel)
A. E. Schindler (West Germany)

INTRODUCTION

Hysterectomy rates have been steadily increasing in Western countries in recent years. (Figures for The Netherlands are given in Table 1.) It has been calculated that if this trend continues, in the near future (a) hysterectomy will become the most frequently performed major surgical procedure in women, and (b) approximately half of all women will lose their uterus at some time of their life (Selwood and Wood, 1978). The reasons for this increase are not exactly clear, but it is possible that the following are among the contributing factors:

(1) The lower surgical risk associated with the procedure, as a consequence of better anaesthesia methods, the prevention and treatment of post-operative infections by antibiotics, and the prevention of thromboembolic complications by the use of anti-coagulants.

(2) A possible increase in the frequency of gynaecological disorders, or perhaps a decrease in the acceptance of minor gynaecological complaints following long-term use of oral or intrauterine methods of contraception.

(3) An expansion of indications for hysterectomy, especially when request for sterilization is combined with minor gynaecological abnormalities or complaints.

(4) An increasing tendency towards preventive medicine: prevention of uterine cancer by elective hysterectomy for sterilization (Cole and Berlin, 1977; Editorial, 1977).

(5) A change in the attitudes of gynaecologists. Selwood and Wood (1978) have formulated this aspect as follows: "Another explanation for the high incidence of hysterectomy may be that the operation is carried out unnecessarily. In this situation, the specialist rationalizes the use of a surgical procedure. Either overtly or subconsciously, the specialist influences the patient towards surgical rather than medical therapy. This would be especially simple in the case of excessive menstrual pain or bleeding. The use of medical therapy in the form of hormone preparations, antiprostaglandins and anti-stress regimes may not be offered to the patient whose choice of treatment may be restricted to curettage or hysterectomy. Hysterectomy is one of the few major operations done by the gynaecologists, and pride, technical practice, and financial incentive may generate a bias towards this treatment."

Table 1 Number of hysterectomies per 100 000 women per year in The Netherlands

1971	254	The increase is most outspoken in the age group 30–34, where the rate rose from 169 per 100 000 women in 1971
1974	311	to 476 in 1979, an increase of 182%, and in the age
1975	329	group 35–39, where it rose from 572 to 1044. Most
1976	346	hysterectomies are performed in women between 40
1977	363	and 50 years of age; in 1979 the rate for this age group
1978	368	was 1440 per 100 000 women.
1979	381	

(Source: SMR-CBS, 1981)

To the moderator of this workshop this 'hysterectomy-boom' is of great concern in view of the reported emotional and sexual disturbances following hysterectomy especially, as might be expected, in the poor indication group. One even might wonder whether another explanation of the eagerness to remove uteri could be that the vast majority of gynaecologists (at least in Western countries) are men, and that hysterectomy represents an unconscious, rationalized act of male aggression and oppression towards femininity. This concern formed the primary incentive to organize this workshop in the hope that more insight might be gained into the background of hysterectomy and of ways in which to prevent unnecessary surgery or, if surgery is necessary, of ways in which to prevent adverse post-hysterectomy sequelae.

EMOTIONAL AND SEXUAL VALUE OF THE UTERUS (Introduced by J. G. van Dijk)

The uterus is traditionally considered to be the centre of femininity and procreation, being an organ that women have and men have not. Even women are not always conscious of having a uterus; its biological expression only becomes really apparent at three phases of their lives: at menarche, during pregnancy, and after menopause. In fact it is only during pregnancy that the uterus becomes an anatomical reality to the woman and her environment. The emotional and sexual value of the uterus is therefore accentuated in situations where the woman never had an uterus (agenesia) or loses one (hysterectomy). The uterus also has emotional and sexual value for men. On one hand they view this organ as something they have not, possibly engendering some kind of 'uterus-envy' comparable to the 'penis-envy' postulated by Freud. An illustration of this is shown in Figure 1, where a rather masculine view of the female genital organs is depicted. On the other hand men also relate the uterus to the origin of human life and to femininity. This intrinsic ambivalence towards the uterus can lead to aggressive feelings (hysterectomy-proneness), but also to feelings of sorrow and bitterness, such as the perception of hysterectomized women as being hollow, empty and no longer feminine. This latter attitude can add to the gravity of post-hysterectomy emotional problems especially because unfortunately women still identify themselves easily with masculine ideas.

It is therefore very important that the gynaecologists (mostly males = 'have nots') be conscious of the fact that their value system concerning the uterus can be different from that of their patients ('haves'). It should be realized that during the decision making process for hysterectomy the uterus can have an emotional value to both patient and gynaecologist, the arguments of the latter in favour of hysterectomy.

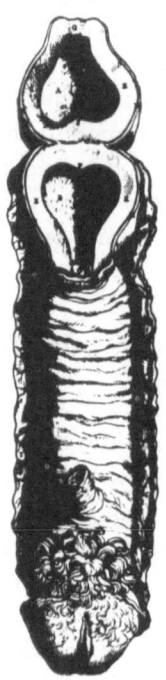

Figure 1   Depiction of female genital organs by Vesalius (1514–1564) for 'Analogi' by Galenus. (Source: E. Fischer-Homberger, *Krankheit-Frau*, 1979.)

PSYCHOSOCIAL, EMOTIONAL AND MEDICAL SEQUELAE OF HYSTERECTOMY (Introduced by B. Ehret and L. Dennerstein)

Ehret spoke of the experiences of approximately 3000 women treated in her institute during the past four years for adverse sequelae after hysterectomy. Most of these women belonged to lower social classes and had a low level of education in general and of sex-education specifically. In 40% of these cases no clear indication for the hysterectomy could be found; there was only a 'relative indication', such as moderate prolapse, ovarian cysts, and small fibroids, to which vague complaints such as abdominal pain, dysmenorrhoea and dyspareunia had been attributed.

87% of the women suffered from so-called post-hysterectomy syndrome: lower abdominal pain, disturbed sexuality, and depression.

It appeared on further investigation that the majority of these women already experienced these complaints before the operation; it seems therefore that the 'post-hysterectomy syndrome' sometimes begins long before the operation, especially in cases where the indication for surgery is poor. Gynaecologists should be aware of this and take time to discover pre-operative psychosomatic problems before recommending a hysterectomy. They should also weigh the indication for hysterectomy against non-surgical alternatives for the treatment of gynaecological complaints such as hypermenorrhoea and pelvic pain which quite often have a psychosomatic background. When there is an indication for hysterectomy pre- and post-operative counselling of the patients, preferably with their partners, is of great importance for the prevention of adverse sequelae. A plea was made for group-counselling sessions of women having undergone hysterectomy (*Cohen*).

Dennerstein has concluded from prospective studies that the likelihood of developing *new* psychiatric problems because of the hysterectomy is probably small, and that most of the psychiatric problems found occur in women who had the same problems pre-operatively.

An interesting hypothesis put forward was that the incidence of post-hysterectomy syndrome would probably be reduced if certain social changes concerning the position of women in society were to occur; if, for instance, there was a de-emphasis on the importance of reproduction for women's self-esteem. The incidence would probably also be reduced if women were to become more knowledgeable about their bodies, and if they were to be more active in their interaction with doctors.

As far as the medical aspects are concerned, it became clear that hysterectomy does not generally affect ovarian function nor does it have any effect on the age of onset of menopause (*Ovadia, Schindler*).

PROPHYLACTIC OOPHORECTOMY AT HYSTERECTOMY (Introduced by P. M. H. G. Buytaert and E. V. van Hall)

The pros and cons of the controversial procedure of castrating women older than 40 years at hysterectomy in order to prevent later ovarian cancer were discussed by, respectively, *Buytaert* and *van Hall*.

The risk of ovarian cancer after hysterectomy varies, according to different retrospective and prospective studies, between 1:100 and 1:1000. This difference in rate is most probably due to differences in the types of studies reported. The relatively high incidence of 1:100 derives from epidemiological studies on the general incidence of ovarian cancer and from retrospective studies where the frequency of previous hysterectomy in women with ovarian cancer has been evaluated (5–10%). In the opinion of the moderator of this workshop these types of data do not give an accurate estimation of the risk of developing ovarian cancer after hysterectomy. The much lower incidence of up to 1:1000 derives from long-term prospective studies in women following hysterectomy (Schweppe and Beller, 1979). There could perhaps even be a place for the hypothesis that hysterectomy protects against the development of later ovarian cancer.

Even if one compromises at the figure of 1 in 500 women developing ovarian cancer after hysterectomy it becomes very much a matter of philosophy and personal attitude: should one castrate 500 women between 40 and 55 years of age in order to prevent *one* ovarian cancer? This decision should be weighed against the personal and general problems arising by the imposition of necessary long-term oestrogen substitution. Such treatment influences the daily quality of life of these women by making them dependent on medical treatment and this, as such, affects their already damaged feeling of normality. Moreover the possible risks of oestrogen substitution, such as increased frequency of cardiovascular disease, must also be taken into account (Centerwall, 1981; Gordon *et al.*, 1978).

DISCUSSION

During the very lively general discussion held at the end of this workshop it appeared that there was a marked sex-difference in the position taken by the participants on the topics discussed, men generally advocating a more aggressive approach and women a more conservative one. In this respect it is interesting to note that of the 8 speakers 4 were women. Male gynaecologists should be more willing to listen to and accept the opinions of their female colleagues as women are more likely to understand the problems related to hysterectomy.

I should like to end this report with a question which seems to me to be of great importance and which was raised during this workshop by Ehret: "What is it that makes such a large number of women allow the prophylactic removal of a healthy organ in the sexual sphere? A similar surgery-boom among men would be unthinkable, because men, as we all know, only undergo an operation when it becomes absolutely necessary.

It is very difficult to find an answer to this question. Actively courageous decisions rarely form the basis for consent to an operation. On the contrary, the decision is often influenced by passive, partly auto-aggressive tendencies. These women view themselves and are viewed by others as sexual objects; they behave in many aspects of life as passive objects and are considered to be physically and psychically inferior. The removal of the uterus from just such a woman is comparable to removing the tear ducts from a crying person''.

References

Centerwall, B. S. (1981). Premenopausal hysterectomy and cardiovascular disease. *Am. J. Obstet. Gynecol.*, **139**, 58

Cole, P. and Berlin, J. (1977). Elective hysterectomy. *Am. J. Obstet. Gynecol.*, **129**, 117

Editorial (1977). Hysterectomy and sterilization: changes of fashion and mind. *Br. Med. J.*, **2**, 715

Gordon, T., Kannel, W. B., Hjortland, M. C. and McNamara, P. M. (1978). Menopause and coronary heart disease. The Framingham Study. *Ann. Intern. Med.*, **89**, 157

Schweppe, K. W. and Beller, F. K. (1979). Zur Frage der prophylaktischen Ovarektomie. *Geburtsh. Frauenheilk.*, **39**, 1024

Selwood, T. and Wood, C. (1978). Incidence of hysterectomy in Australia. *Med. J. Aust.*, **2**, 201

Workshop 9

Androgens in post-menopausal women

Moderator: **A. Vermeulen** (Belgium)

Speakers: **J. Botella Llusiá** (Spain)
V. H. T. James (UK)
R. Lindsay (USA)
J. Poortman (The Netherlands)
A. Vermeulen (Belgium)

SEX HORMONE LEVELS IN POST-MENOPAUSAL WOMEN
(Introduced by A. Vermeulen)

In post-menopausal women the adrenal cortex is the main source of all sex hormones. It is true that after the menopause the ovaries continue to secrete testosterone, and in some cases (Longcope has estimated the figure to be around 20%) also minute amounts of oestrogens. Most oestrogens found in post-menopausal women however come from the adrenal cortex, not through direct secretion but from the peripheral conversion of androgens.

Androstenedione appears to be the most important precursor of plasma oestrogen – the concentration of which is largely determined by the precursor concentration and by fat mass, the latter being a very important determinant of plasma oestrogen levels.

Age seems to affect adrenal cortical androgen secretion, but whereas the plasma levels of Δ5 steroid show a highly significant age-dependent decrease, androstenedione and more generally Δ4 plasma steroid levels do not change much with age. Similarly, the response to short-term ACTH stimulation shows a difference between the Δ5 steroids, the response of which decreases with age, and the Δ4 steroids, where no age-related change is seen. The factors which determine this ageing of the adrenal cortex remain to be elucidated. It seems unlikely, however, that changes in oestrogen or in prolactin levels play a rôle. Indeed, oestrogen therapy remains without influence in this respect, and while in post-menopausal women the decrease of adrenal Δ5 steroid secretion occurs at a time when the prolactin levels are depressed, in males the same adrenal ageing phenomena occur at a time when the prolactin levels are raised.

OVARIAN CONTRIBUTION TO SEX HORMONE LEVELS IN POST-MENOPAUSAL WOMEN (Introduced by J. Botella Llusiá)

Botella Llusiá has studied ovarian sex hormone secretion in post-menopausal women by direct catheterization of the ovarian vein. He has observed that the post-menopausal ovary continues to produce testosterone, probably in greater quantities than during reproductive life. Using this method of investigation *Botella Llusiá* has further found higher testosterone levels in patients with adenocarcinoma of the endometrium and whenever there was a proliferative endometrium, but no evidence of any increase in the ovarian secretion of oestrogen. It would seem, therefore, that the high levels of peripheral oestrogen found in patients with endometrial adenocarcinoma or a proliferative endometrium do indeed come not from the ovary but from a peripheral conversion of androgen.

SEX HORMONES AND POST-MENOPAUSAL OSTEOPOROSIS (Introduced by R. Lindsay)

Lindsay has studied the rate of endogenous steroid production in accelerated post-menopausal osteoporosis. In a series of studies he has shown that bone loss is related to cortisol production, as well as to circulating oestrogen and androgen levels. A dynamic study of adrenal function, however, could not determine any difference between women losing bone and those who were not, when $\Delta 4$ and $\Delta 5$ steroid production was followed after ACTH stimulation. In these relatively young post-menopausal women (aged 40–60 years) *Lindsay* and his co-workers found some evidence of lower circulating levels of androstenedione and oestrone both in oophorectomized women and in those who were losing bone fastest, together with a gradual fall with age. They have not, however, found the sudden fall in androstenedione levels that has been described elsewhere and which is sometimes referred to as 'the adreno-pause'. There is no doubt that more rapid bone loss in the early post-menopausal years is associated both with low circulating androstene-dione levels and with low total oestrogen levels (measured as oestradiol plus oestrone). Recently *Lindsay* has noted that mestranol therapy appears to increase androstenedione levels in oophorectomized women, without a significant change in cortisol production. Clearly further investigation of the rôle of the adrenal androgens and of other adrenal steroids in post-menopausal bone loss is an area which may well provide useful information in the future.

The fact that oestrogens play an aetiological rôle in osteoporosis is proven by the clear-cut and long-lasting therapeutic effects of oestrogen treatment, which decreases or arrests the rate of bone loss; this has been shown by *Lindsay*, using a variety of parameters, and in cases followed for up to 10 years. A good parameter of the rate of bone loss appears to be the retention of diphosphonates 24 h after administration, retention being inversely related to bone loss. It appears that the minimal thera-peutic dose required is between 0.3 and 0.6 mg conjugated equine oestrogens/day, a comparatively low dose which may be considered a relatively safe one. Interestingly, calcium supplements 1.5 g/day seem to be almost as effective.

As to the mechanism of action of oestrogens, much remains to elucidated. Both parathormone and calcitonin levels rise during oestrogen therapy, and oestrogen may promote the hydroxylation of vitamin D. An interesting finding is that in patients with a high rate of bone loss, urinary free cortisol excretion is increased. Whether or not this is a consequence of a lower transcortin level, itself the consequence of lower oestrogen levels, is not yet clear. Finally, *Lindsay* reported that a controlled study of an anabolic agent (OD14) has recently confirmed that steroid agents other than oestrogens may also effectively prevent bone loss without inducing endometrial growth. OD14 may well prove of great interest in the future as its side effects appear to be minimal.

ADRENAL ANDROGEN PRODUCTION IN MAMMARY AND ENDOMETRIAL CANCER (Introduced by J. Poortman and V. H. T. James respectively)

Several pieces of evidence suggest that oestrogens play an important rôle in determining a hormonal environment which favours the development of mammary and of endometrial cancer. For example, (a) epidemiological studies show that increased oestrogen production is associated with an increase in risk, while diminished production is associated with a decrease in risk, (b) the influence of weight as a risk factor may be explained by the increased conversion in heavier women of androgens into oestrogens, (c) the administration of oestrogens to post-menopausal women is said to increase the risk of endometrial cancer, and finally (d) oestrogens increase the growth rate of mammary cancer cells in culture.

As adrenal androgens are the major source of circulating oestrogens in post-menopausal women, it is of interest to study adrenal androgen secretion in patients with mammary or endometrial cancer. The well-known, almost historical, data of Bulbrook showing a decreased urinary androgen excretion in mammary cancer patients have been confirmed. On the other hand, when expressed per unit of creatinine, 11-desoxo-17-keto-steroid excretion has been found to be similar in cancerous and in non-cancerous patients. *Poortman* has therefore concluded that the determination of androgen metabolite excretion in women over 50 years of age is of no help in selecting a group of women at high risk of developing breast cancer. Furthermore, he has observed no differences in plasma levels of androgens, be they dehydroepiandrosterone, its sulphate, testosterone, or their total, between patients with breast cancer and age-matched controls, nor any significant differences in androstenedione or dehydroepiandrosterone (sulphate) production rates. Moreover, the conversion of androstenedione to oestrone was not significantly increased in women with breast cancer.

Poortman has not yet been able to define a particular hormone profile that is associated with an increased risk of mammary cancer. It may well be that the methods available at present are too crude to detect subtle differences. It is probable however that the measurement of receptor and hormone levels in target tissues and their subcellular distribution will one day permit a better understanding of the rôle of hormone factors in the aetiology of this disease.

As the plasma concentration of a hormone represents the balance between its production and its clearance, *James* investigated whether

84

differences exist in production and clearance of androgens and of oestrogens between women with cancer and normal controls. As far as plasma levels and androgen (dehydroepiandrosterone, its sulphate, and androstenedione) and of oestrogen (oestrone and oestradiol) were concerned, he found no significant differences between mammary cancer patients and normal controls matched for age and weight, although in patients with breast cancer, unbound oestradiol levels tended to be higher than in weight-matched controls. It was observed that in normal post-menopausal women the metabolic clearance rate of oestrone and of oestradiol was 30% lower than in younger women, but that in patients with endometrial carcinoma or hyperplasia it was higher. The major determinant of this increase, however, appeared to be weight. Production rates of oestrone and of oestradiol similarly appeared to be higher in women with endometrial carcinoma, but again this appeared to be determined by weight. Hence, in agreement with Siiteri and MacDonald, *James* found an increased oestrogen production in some patients with endometrial cancer. As progesterone levels are extremely low in post-menopausal women, and as progesterone is known to modulate tissue oestradiol concentration, it could well be that this increased oestrogen production has profound effects on endometrial tissue.

James feels that an important point requiring further investigation is the observation that although oestrone is a major source of oestradiol in post-menopausal women, it seems that a substantial amount of oestradiol may be derived from other, as yet unidentified, sources. These sources could include direct ovarian or adrenal secretion. It is also possible, however, that conjugated androgens, androstenedione sulphate for example, play a rôle as prehormones. Androstenedione is an important precursor for oestrone, but the factors influencing aromatase and 17β-reductase activity are not yet apparent. It is possible that progesterone plays a rôle as a modulating agent. It is clear though that adipose tissue is not homogeneous biochemically, and it may be that local tissue activity, as yet undisclosed in overall kinetic studies, is of considerable biological and clinical significance.

CONCLUDING COMMENTS

It is clear that much work has still to be done before we can expect to have a good insight into the complicated interrelationships between mammary and endometrial cancer and adrenal cortical hormone secretion and metabolism. Other lines of research which may well be helpful are studies of the rôle of adrenal steroids in modulating hormone action and metabolism at the tissular level, and a systematic study of factors which affect the binding of hormones to testosterone-oestradiol binding globulin, an important determinant of tissue exposure to active hormones.

Bibliography

Botella Llusiá, J., Oriol Bosch, A., Sánchez Garrido, F. and Tresguerres, J. A. F. (1980). Testosterone and 17β-oestradiol secretion of the human ovary. II. Normal postmenopausal women, postmenopausal women with endometrial hyperplasia, and postmenopausal women with adenocarcinoma of the endometrium. *Maturitas*, **2**, 7

Deslypere, J. P. and Vermeulen, A. (1981). Aging and tissue androgens. *J. Clin. Endocrinol. Metab.*, **53**, 430

Drafta, D., Schindler, A. E., Milcu, St. M., Keller, E., Stroe, E., Horodniceanu, E. and Balanescu, I. (1980). Plasma hormones in pre- and post-menopausal breast cancer. *J. Steroid Biochem.*, **13**, 793

James, V. H. T. and Reed, M. J. (1980). Steroid hormones and human cancer. In Iacobelli, S., King, R. J. B., Lindner, H. R. and Lippman, M. E. (eds.) *Hormones and Cancer*, p. 471. (New York: Raven Press)

Judd, H. L., Davidson, B. J., Frumar, A. M., Shamonki, I. M., Lagasse, L. D. and Ballon, S. C. (1980). Serum androgens and estrogens in post-menopausal women with and without endometrial cancer. *Am. J. Obstet. Gynec.*, **136**, 859

Lindsay, R., Hart, D. M., Aitken, J. M., MacDonald, E. B., Anderson, J. B. and Clark, A. (1976). Long-term prevention of postmenopausal osteoporosis by oestrogen. *Lancet*, **1**, 1038

Lindsay, R., Hart, D. M., Forrest, C. and Baird, C. (1980). Prevention of spinal osteoporosis in oophorectomised women. *Lancet*, **2**, 1151

Lindsay, R., Hart, D. M. and Kraszewski, A. (1980). Prospective double-blind trial of a synthetic steroid (Org OD14) for preventing postmenopausal osteoporosis. *Br. Med. J.*, **280**, 1207

Poortman, J. (1980). Role of steroid hormones in the genesis of human mammary cancer. *Reviews on Endocrine-related Cancer*, nr. 6, 27

Poortman, J. and Thijssen, J. H. H. (1978). The role of androgens in the aetiology of endometrial cancer – a hypothesis. In Brush, M. G., King, R. J. B. and Taylor, R. W. (eds.) *Endometrial Cancer*, pp. 375–382. (London: Baillière Tindall)

Siiteri, P. K. (1981). Extraglandular estrogen formation and serum binding of estradiol: relationship to cancer. *J. Endocrinol.*, **89**, 119

Siiteri, P. K., Nisker, J. A. and Hammond, G. L. (1980). Hormonal basis of risk factors for breast and endometrial cancer. In Iacobelli, S., King, R. J. B., Lindner, H. R. and Lippman, M. E. (eds.) *Hormones and Cancer*, p. 499 (New York: Raven Press)

Vermeulen, A. and Verdonck, L. (1978). Sex hormone concentrations in postmenopausal women. *Clin. Endocrinol.*, **9**, 59

Workshop 10

The peri-menopause at the cellular level

Moderator: **J. H. H. Thijssen** (The Netherlands)

Speakers: **F. Bayard** (France)
E. W. Bergink (The Netherlands)
M. van Haaften (The Netherlands)
R. J. B. King (UK)
J. R. Pasqualini (France)
N. C. Siddle (UK)
L. Tseng (USA)
M. A. H. M. Wiegerinck (The Netherlands)

INTRODUCTION

There were several possible ways of dealing with the subject of this workshop. The central theme finally chosen was the mechanism of action of steroid hormones, attention being paid not only to oestrogens, but also to progestational substances. The questions raised at the beginning of the session were:

(1) What do we know about the way in which steroids act at the cellular level?
(2) What do we know about the handling *in vivo* of oestrogens by target tissues in post-menopausal women?
(3) Is it possible to identify and to quantitate specific effects of steroid interactions with tissues?
(4) Are we able to relate some of these specific effects to clinically important events?

MECHANISM OF ACTION OF STEROID HORMONES

The starting point of the discussion was the supposed mechanism of action of steroid hormones. This is illustrated for oestradiol in Figure 1.

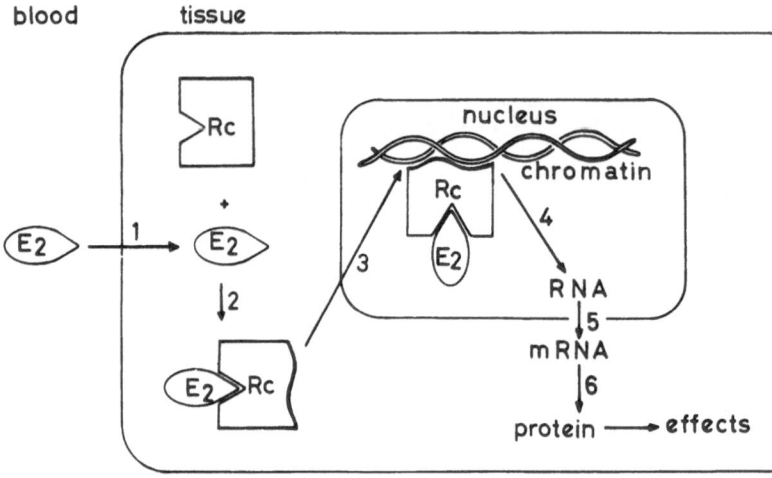

Figure 1   The supposed mechanism of action of oestradiol. The following steps can be distinguished: 1, Passive transport of the steroid through the cell membrane; 2, Its binding to the intracellular receptor, resulting in the transformation of the protein; 3, The translocation of the steroid receptor complex to the nucleus, and its binding to chromatin; 4, Synthesis of RNA; 5, Increase in mRNA in the cytosol; 6, Protein synthesis, and occurrence of specific effects (E_2=oestradiol, Rc=receptor)

In order to act on any tissue the steroid has first to be taken up by the cell (step 1). According to recent literature, this uptake takes place without any particular active process occurring, but simply by direct diffusion (Müller and Wotiz, 1979). Upon arrival in the cells of the target tissue, the steroid binds to a specific binding protein, in this example, to the oestrogen receptor; this binding results in the transformation of the receptor molecule (step 2). Following this transformation, and only then, the steroid receptor complex is translocated to the nucleus of the cell (step 3), where it binds to the chromatin. This binding induces the production of RNA (ribonucleic acid) (step 4), which results in an increase in mRNA (messenger RNA) in the cytoplasma (step 5), and subsequently in effects on the synthesis of specific proteins (step 6). It is suspected, but not yet confirmed, that the effect of oestrogens on cell proliferation is mediated by steps 4–6.

One of the specific effects of oestrogens at the cellular level is the induction of progesterone receptors.

The mechanism of action of progesterone on cells is very similar to that described above for oestrogens. The interaction of progestational substances with the progesterone receptors also results in specific effects, one of which is the induction of the enzyme 17β-hydroxy steroid dehydrogenase which is capable of converting oestradiol into oestrone and *vice versa*; within the cells the equilibrium is in the direction of oestrone, which means that in the presence of this dehydrogenase the intracellular oestradiol concentration decreases.

UPTAKE AND HANDLING *IN VIVO* OF OESTROGENS

In the first contribution to this workshop *Wiegerinck* reported on his *in vivo* studies under physiological conditions of the uptake and metabolism of oestrone, oestradiol and oestriol in post-menopausal endometrial, myometrial and vaginal tissues. His studies of the distribution and concentrations in subcellular fractions have shown clear differences in the uptake of individual oestrogens by the tissues; oestradiol and oestriol accumulated similarly in the nuclei of the target cells in concentrations at least 10 times greater than in plasma, whereas almost no tissue:plasma gradient could be found for oestrone. In addition to the differences found between the three oestrogens studied, differences were also observed between the three tissues investigated. In all patients the tissue:plasma gradients of oestradiol and of oestriol in the endometrium and myometrium were greater than in the vagina. Although histologically the endometria were all classified as atrophic, the endometrial cells were clearly very active in building up a large gradient to plasma for some oestrogens. A number of conclusions of clinical relevance can be drawn from these studies:

(1) Oestrogen concentrations in target cells are completely different from those found in plasma.
(2) Oestradiol is the most important tissue-oestrogen in post-menopausal women, as well as in younger women.
(3) Oestrone can be considered as merely a pre-hormone, a precursor for oestradiol.
(4) Biochemically measured, an atrophic endometrium is more active than the vagina in concentrating oestradiol.
(5) Factors which influence the equilibrium *in vivo* between oestrone and oestradiol in the circulation are largely unknown.

SPECIFIC BINDING PROTEINS

Following its uptake by the cell, the steroid has to bind to a specific binding protein; for oestradiol it is oestrogen receptor. Some evidence has recently been found that not all oestrogen binding proteins have exactly the same characteristics. *Bayard* described his findings in this connection. Starting from the observation that in the human MCF-7 cell line there is an influence of anti-oestrogens on cells but no oestrogen receptors, *Bayard*'s studies led to the discovery of a protein to which several anti-oestrogens specifically bind. He has been able to demonstrate the existence of such a protein in several human tissues, namely the endometrium, myometrium and fibromyomata. It appears that the anti-oestrogen protein complex is able to interfere in some way with the oestrogen receptor complex in the nucleus. The concentration of the anti-oestrogen binding protein is not related to the oestrogen receptor concentration. It is completely unknown at the present time whether a naturally occurring steroid exists which acts via this binding protein; the physiological rôle of this protein is therefore open to speculation.

Bergink also reported on the existence of a binding protein which is completely different from the known oestrogen receptors. This is a protein which has a high affinity specifically for oestriol, and which has been found in the vagina of post-menopausal women after several weeks' administration of oestriol. *Bergink* described the binding characteristics of this protein, but here too it is not yet possible to say anything about any physiological or pharmacological rôle which this protein might have.

It was clear from the first part of this workshop that there very probably are proteins in the human target tissue cells which are able to bind oestrogens and anti-oestrogens, but which are different from the known oestradiol receptors. It seems that these binding proteins interfere with the expected actions of oestrogens at the cellular level, but their rôle and their importance are not yet understood.

EFFECTS OF STEROID RECEPTOR INTERACTIONS

The second part of the workshop dealt with the (specific) effects of oestrogens and of progesterone. It became clear from the various contributions that these effects are divergent. This implies that, at least in part, the specificity of the tissue responses is caused by differences in the intranuclear handling of the steroid receptor complexes, as such divergency cannot be explained simply by differences in the binding of the steroids to the specific receptors. In particular, cell proliferation and multiplication are stimulated in a way different from the biochemically measurable effects.

Van Haaften drew attention to the fact that one does not find measurable amounts of progestogen receptors in the vagina; one would normally have expected to do so, since the vagina is highly responsive to oestrogens, and the induction of progestogen receptors is, or was, regarded as one of the specific effects of oestrogen in target cells.

The reactions of steroid metabolizing enzymes to progesterone and synthetic progestational substances in the human endometrium were reported by *Tseng*. It became apparent from her presentation that it is necessary to separate the effects in the glandular from those in the stromal compartment of the endometrium as the location of the enzymes investigated shows clear discrepancies: the concentration of 17-OHSD (17β-hydroxy-steroid-oxidoreductase), which converts oestradiol into oestrone and *vice versa*, is some 2–3 times higher in glandular epithelial cells than in stromal cells, and the oestrogen-sulphotransferase, which converts oestrone and oestradiol to their 17-sulphates, is almost exclusively present in the epithelial cells. Stimulation of 17-OHSD by different progestational substances parallels the binding of these substances to the progesterone receptor. The influence of progesterone on the action of oestrogens on the endometrium cannot simply be explained by the influence of progesterone on the metabolism of oestrogens in the endometrial cells.

Although the increase in oestradiol metabolizing enzymes is of importance, the conclusion must be that the anti-oestrogenic effects of progestins on the human endometrium are more complicated to explain.

The need to separate the hormonal effects on stromal from those on the glandular cells was also stressed by *King*. As an example, he showed that after oestrogen stimulation the increase in the number of progesterone receptors was much greater in the epithelial than in the stromal cells. The post-menopausal endometria used in this study were obtained from patients after treatment with conjugated oestrogens with or without norethisterone. Regarding the effects of these treatments, a good correlation was found between the amount of nuclear oestrogen receptor and the [3H]thymidine incorporation, chosen as a parameter for cell replication activity. From the biochemically measurable effects it can be concluded that treatments with progestational substances following oestrogen administration should be given for at least six days before clear results can be expected to be seen on the endometrium.

Pasqualini agreed with what had been said by the other speakers regarding the divergency of effects at the cellular level. He reported that in the fetal guinea-pig uterus he found stimulation with oestradiol to result in far greater effect than oestriol on growth, whereas the effect of the two oestrogens on the induction of progesterone receptors was very similar.

Finally, *Siddle* reported on the *in vivo* effects of the anti-oestrogen tamoxifen compared with those of the progestagen norgestrel on the human uterus after pre-treatment with conjugated oestrogens. With the exception of the fact that both treatments had a similar depressing effect on DNA-synthesis (measured by [^{3}H]thymidine incorporation), the two treatments had different effects on all the parameters measured, i.e., on the accumulation of the nuclear oestrogen receptors, on the induction of the progesterone receptors, and on 17-OHSD and isocitric dehydrogenase activity.

It can be concluded from all these contributions that different treatments will clearly have demonstrable diverging effects on the human endometrium. It is also clear that in all studies in the future the differences between the stromal and the epithelial cells of uterine tissue must be taken into account.

CONCLUSIONS AND RECOMMENDATIONS

Summarizing the subjects dealt with during this workshop, a number of relevant conclusions may be drawn:

(1) The concentration of steroid hormones in the target tissues is different from those in blood, even when protein binding of hormones is taken into account.

(2) Besides the specific oestrogen receptor, other binding proteins with different and specific binding characteristics are present in some organs; their rôle and their importance are unclear at the moment.

(3) A difference can be demonstrated between endometrium, myometrium and vagina regarding the uptake and cellular handling of oestrogens.

(4) The tissue handling of the three 'classical' oestrogens – oestrone, oestradiol and oestriol – is not identical; oestrone may be considered as a pre-hormone of the more active oestradiol.

(5) Effects which have previously been thought to be specific as an effect of hormonal action should not be considered to be specific in all tissues without prior proof.

(6) Oestrogens and progestins have a number of biological effects which can be quantified biochemically. A clear divergence of effects has been demonstrated, especially between stimulation of replication and induction of receptors and/or enzymes.

(7) It is evident that our knowledge regarding the mechanism of action of oestrogens and of progestins has improved greatly of late. We now have techniques which enable us to measure both receptors and some effects of steroid receptor interactions. In the future, studies should attempt to relate clinical observations and biochemical findings to each other. When doing so, attention should be paid not only to cytoplasmic receptor concentrations, but also to steroid levels in tissue, to nuclear receptor concentrations, and to measurable specific effects of cell activation.

Bibliography

King, R. J. B., Whitehead, M. I., Campbell, S. and Minardi, J. (1979). Effect of estrogen and progestin treatments on endometria from postmenopausal women. *Cancer Res.*, **39**, 1094

Müller, R. E. and Wotiz, H. H. (1979). Kinetics of estradiol entry into uterine cells. *Endocrinology*, **105**, 1107

Pasqualini, J. R., Gulino, A., Nguyen, B. L. and Portois, M. C. (1980). Receptor and biological response to estriol in the fetal uterus of guinea pig. *J. Receptor Res.*, **1**, 261

Sutherland, R. L. and Murphy, L. C. (1980). The binding of tamoxifen to human mammary carcinoma cytosol. *Eur. J. Cancer*, **16**, 1141

Thijssen, J. H. H., Wiegerinck, M. H. A. M., Mulder, G. and Poortman, J. (1978). On the biological activity of estrone *in vivo*. In Lauritzen, C. and van Keep, P. A. (eds.) *Estrogen Therapy – the Benefits and Risks. Front. Hormone Res.*, Vol. 5, pp. 220–229. (Basel: Karger)

Tseng, L. (1980). Hormonal regulation of steroid metabolic enzymes in human endometrium. In Thomas, J. A. and Singhai, R. L. (eds.) *Advances in Sex Hormone Research.* Vol. IV, pp. 329–361 (Baltimore and Munich: Urban and Schwarzenberg)

Workshop 11

Osteoporosis

Moderator: **O. L. M. Bijvoet** (The Netherlands)

Speakers: **R. P. Heaney** (USA)
G. Milhaud (France)
B. E. C. Nordin (UK)
B. L. Riggs (USA)

There is certainly much controversy around the subject of osteoporosis. The noise associated with frontline battles may obscure perception of very real acquisitions that have been made in areas of practical significance. The importance of therapy – of treatments with calcium, oestrogens, fluoride, and possibly vitamin D – is now less disputed and deserves to be more generally appreciated. Four authors, each with much experience in this field, were invited to participate in this workshop and to enlarge upon those issues which they considered to be of greatest importance. Their contributions are summarized in this report.

The first speaker was *Nordin*, who spoke on the controversial matter of the mechanism of the development of osteoporosis. He presented a new model to explain, in quantitative terms, the regulation of trabecular bone volume, in terms of the forming and resorbing activity. This is important, because at the present time there is no agreement as to the extent to which reduced bone formation, increased bone resorption, or a combination of the two, is responsible for age-related bone loss (simple osteoporosis) or for the crush fracture syndrome (accelerated osteoporosis).

Nordin's group has analysed quantitative histological data from 522 iliac crest bone biopsies in several conditions. In young women bone-forming surfaces were found to be unrelated to total surfaces but resorbing surfaces were highly correlated with total surfaces. This is related to the concept, which appears to apply in many biological circumstances, that quantities are often regulated by equilibrium between a linear influx rate (quantity per unit of time) and a fractional efflux (fraction per unit of time). Starting from an equilibrium situation, any permanent change of influx or efflux is translated as a transient change of total quantity until equilibrium is again obtained, at the moment that fractional removal (f) times quantity $(Q$ units) equals addition $(a$, units per time)

$$a = f.Q$$

According to this concept the total quantity of trabecular bone is considered directly proportional to the ratio between forming activity (mean number of osteoid covered surfaces per microscopic field) and resorbtive activity (resorbing surfaces as a fraction, or percentage, of total surfaces). A comparison of young and old female control data and female osteoporotics showed that the age-related bone loss in women is a function of increased bone resorption only; there was no difference in the mean forming surfaces of the two groups. When elderly normal women were compared with osteoporotic women, resorbing activity was significantly reduced.

In males the picture is different. Age-related bone loss is entirely accounted for by a decline in forming surfaces, but when osteoporotic and normal elderly men are compared the osteoporosis in the former is entirely accounted for by increased resorption.

This concept explains why trabecular bone loss in normal subjects is self-limiting. In both sexes, though for different reasons, there is a decline in bone volume in the sixth decade with no significant decline thereafter.

Nordin considers that the increased bone resorption in the male and female osteoporotic subjects is probably attributable to malabsorption of calcium.

At the same time, however, the menopause is associated with a rise in plasma and urinary calcium, in phosphate levels, and in plasma alkaline phosphatase and urinary hydroxyproline. All these changes can be reversed with oestrogen therapy in the usual 'replacement' doses. There appears to be no change in calcium absorption at the menopause, nor does calcium absorption change when oestrogen therapy is given.

The biochemical changes observed can be attributed to an increased sensitivity of bone to the resorbing actions of parathyroid hormone and of $1,25\text{-}(OH)_2D_3$ when oestrogen levels fall, expressed, at the histological level, as an increase in the fraction of resorption surface. Kinetic measurements indicate that oestrogen therapy reduces resorption more than formation and improves calcium balance by a mean value of 1 mmol/day, with a similar reduction in urine calcium.

The negative calcium balance of the post-menopausal woman can be regarded as an increase in calcium requirement. The rise in urine calcium at the menopause causes a disproportionate rise in requirement because of a non-linear relation between calcium intake and absorbed calcium. Consequently the requirement of post-menopausal women with normal absorption is 1200 mg/day.

Long-term sequential bone measurements are compatible with complete inhibition of bone loss with oestrogen therapy and considerable reduction with calcium supplements in normal women. The effects are additive. Malabsorption, which is not generally associated with low plasma levels of $25\text{-}(OH)D_3$ or $1,25\text{-}(OH)_2D_3$, responds to treatment with 10 000 units of vitamin D, $20\text{-}40\,\mu g$ 25-OHD, or $1\text{-}2\,\mu g$ 1αD. The simultaneous use of oestrogens or, if oestrogens are contraindicated, of norethisterone appears to entirely obviate the ensuing risk of increased bone resorption or hypercalcaemia.

Identifying women at risk is still a problem. Risk factors seem to include malabsorption of calcium and low plasma oestrogen levels, a high fasting urinary calcium and hydroxyproline, and a high normal plasma alkaline phosphatase. In addition, osteoporotic patients have a significantly thinner skin than age-matched controls, but whether this measurement has predictive value is uncertain.

Riggs reviewed the value of fluoride treatment for osteoporosis. This treatment was first used in 1961 by Rich and Ensinck, who reasoned that the induction of subclinical fluorosis might strengthen the skeleton but not lead to other changes. There is now growing consensus about the effect of fluoride therapy on bone. The predominant effect is to increase bone formation, but chronic ingestion impairs mineralization; however, unlike usual osteomalacia, mineralized bone mass increases, and adverse changes can be minimized by supplementary dietary calcium. The net effect of this treatment is to increase bone mass in the axial skeleton. *Riggs* and his group have tried to answer the following questions, all of which should be resolved before fluoride and calcium regimen can be recommended for unrestricted use:

(1) *Does long-term therapy decrease the occurrence of vertebral fractures? Riggs* and his co-workers have evaluated the fracture incidence in 36 patients with primary osteoporosis treated for up to six years with sodium fluoride, calcium supplements, and, in 24 patients, with vitamin D. New vertebral fractures occurred at the rate of 329 fractures per 1000 years of observation. This is less than half of the expected fracture rate. 45% of the fractures occurred during the first year of therapy. The authors conclude that one year of therapy is insufficient to reduce the fracture rate substantially, but that thereafter the decrease in the fracture rate is striking.

(2) *Is long-term treatment safe?* In published series significant side effects have been reported in one-third to one-half of patients. Rheumatic symptoms (synovitis or painful plantar fascial syndrome) occurred in 11 of the 36 patients in the above-mentioned series and gastrointestinal symptoms (blood loss, anaemia and recurrent vomiting) occurred in 7. Symptoms disappeared upon discontinuation of therapy and did not recur when therapy was reinstituted at a lower dose level.

(3) *What dose of sodium fluoride should be used?* There is no definite answer. At doses below 40 mg/day poor responses may occur and at those above 90 mg/day histological osteomalacia may be seen. *Riggs* and his co-workers recommend 60 mg/day NaF combined with 1.0 to 1.5 g calcium.

(4) *Is there a differential effect on trabecular and cortical bone?* Photon absorption densitometry of the distal radius performed in 16 patients was unchanged in *Riggs*'s series, but in 12 of these 16 patients there was radiographic evidence of an increase in vertebral bone density. It was suggested that the increase in bone mass is largely limited to trabecular bone of the axial skeleton.

(5) *What factors account for differences in individual responsiveness?* In 16 of 28 patients there was no radiographic evidence of increased vertebral bone density and in 12 there was. The fracture rate in the first 16 continued at 536 per 1000 years, the 12 others fractured at the rate of 91 per 1000 years. Prior to treatment the fracture rates of the two groups did not differ. Doses and mean serum levels of fluoride did not differ. The investigators suggest that an intrinsic defect of osteoblasts may limit responsiveness in some osteoporotic patients.

Riggs also reported preliminary results on the anti-fracture efficacy of various combination regimes. The fracture rate in an untreated population of osteoporotic women has been estimated to be more than 800 per 1000 years. Treatment with calcium and vitamin D reduces this to 400–500. The addition of NaF to calcium and vitamin D diminishes the rate still further to 200–300 per 1000 years, and similar results are obtained when oestrogens are combined with calcium and vitamin D. The preliminary results further suggest that a combination of fluoride, calcium, vitamin D and oestrogens – a treatment observed in 28 patients for 113 observation years – would result in a reduction of the fracture rate to figures as low as 25–50 per 1000 years.

Milhaud recalled that it was Fuller Albright at the Massachusetts General Hospital who first related osteoporosis in women to the menopause and who suggested that a lack of oestrogen was responsible for the bone disease. He reminded the audience that there are no oestrogen receptors in bone, and that oestrogens fail to inhibit bone destruction *in vitro*. In his opinion the mechanism of action of oestrogens in this respect, if any, is, to say the least, unclear. *Milhaud* also queried the efficacy of calcium supplements in osteoporosis. He then drew attention to the rôle played by his group in France in the discovery of calcitonin and in the elucidation of its various physiological effects. The most well-known of these is an inhibition of bone resorption, with a subsequent lowering of serum calcium. It has been postulated that the major actions of calcitonin are related to calcium metabolism, as are those of parathyroid hormone and of $1,25\text{-}(OH)_2D_3$.

Calcitonin can be assayed by radioimmunological methods. It is secreted in excess in medullary cancer of the thyroid, which is a cancer of calcitonin-secreting cells. The definite physiological significance of calcitonin is not yet clear. Some authors consider it to be a calcium- or bone-sparing hormone.

Data from Professor MacIntyre's laboratory (at the Postgraduate Medical School in London) suggest intricate relationships between oestrogen and calcitonin metabolism. Both groups, that of *MacIntyre* and that of *Milhaud*, have suggested that post-menopausal osteoporosis is associated with a deficiency of calcitonin leading to an insufficient inhibition of bone destruction. This theory led *Milhaud* to try the administration of physiological doses of calcitonin as substitutive treatment of osteoporosis. One striking observation, which has also been reported in other studies in which calcitonin has been used, even though authors have not always been able to detect objective evidence of improvement in other aspects, is a partial alleviation of bone pain. Since *Milhaud*'s group started this treatment they have found that analysis of the results, taking into account multiple factors, such as alleviation of pain and change of calcium balance, indicates that the therapy is a good one. This treatment with low-dose calcitonin is now widely used in France, but the French findings have yet to be confirmed by workers in other countries. At the present time it must be said that evidence of the value of calcitonin in the treatment of osteoporosis is less soundly based than that relating to treatment with oestrogens and with calcium.

Heaney discussed the problem of the identification of patients at risk. He confirmed that it appears reasonably well established that age-related loss of cortical bone in post-menopausal women can be largely prevented by oestrogen prophylaxis, and that oestrogens reduce the fracture risk as well as maintain skeletal mass. In a later discussion the recommended dose was given as 10 to 15 μg ethinyloestradiol and 1 g elemental calcium. Some authors add progestogens because of their known protective action. When oestrogens are contraindicated *Nordin* uses 5 mg norethisterone, though this appears somewhat less effective than oestrogen. Since the beneficial effect of oestrogen in retarding age-related bone loss is counterbalanced by fear of possible risk, it is important to identify those most likely to develop osteoporotic fracture so as not needlessly to expose individuals who may never have been at risk in the first place. Indeed, given the likelihood of effective prophylaxis, the identification of those at risk may well be the most important practical issue in the field today.

Features that are currently considered to be markers of a risk for osteo-porotic fracture include a low peak bone mass at 35 years of age, small body size, a fair complexion, thin skin, sparse body hair and a positive family history. Nevertheless it is clear that osteoporotic fractures occur in persons who do not fit this profile, and the best that can be said is that these features are more likely to be found in osteoporotic women than in non-osteoporotics of similar age. In addition to the factors mentioned above, which may be said to be related to genetic predisposition, there are other factors which are known to increase risk; these include a sedentary life style, a low calcium intake, or an intake inadequate for needs, as is found, for instance, in people using aluminium hydroxide, who have a vegetarian diet or one over-rich in protein fibre, or who are alcoholics. Further adverse effects are suggested to be a high caffeine intake and smoking. Additional risks are associated with early meno-pause, mast cell dysfunction, and chronic acidosis. In a large population study (by Christiansen) the plasma oestradiol level was found to be an inverse function of bone loss.

It is reasonably well established that in any age cohort fractures are concentrated in those with the least bone mass. The Singh index has been shown to predict for hip fracture, as has the size of the calcar femorale. Trabecular bone volume on iliac crest biopsy is negatively correlated with propensity to crush fracture of the vertebrae. Hence, reduced bone mass, using suitable index bones, is probably a reliable indicator of fracture risk. Unfortunately it is applicable only after the damage (reduced bone mass) has been done, and so does not help to select women for prophylactic oestrogen therapy. *Heaney* and his co-workers have started a 20-year prospective study of 200 normal women, designed to identify predictive factors. The study was begun while subjects were at a clearly pre-osteoporotic peri-menopausal stage. Until fractures occur it will not be possible to determine which, if any, of the features measured will prove to have predictive value.

In addition to what had been said by previous authors, *Heaney* mentioned that at the menopause calcium absorption becomes less effective and urinary calcium conservation less. This leads to a negative calcium balance. The relation between calcium intake and balance is then such that equilibrium balance is only obtained at intakes around 1.4 g elemental calcium/day. Use of oestrogens shifts the line relating balance to intake upwards, so that equilibrium balances are already obtained at intakes of around 1 g calcium/day.

Workshop 12

Potency and hepato-cellular effects of oestrogens after oral, percutaneous, and subcutaneous administration

Moderator: **S. Campbell** (UK)

Secretary: **M. I. Whitehead** (UK)

Speakers: **P. F. Brenner** (USA)
F. Elkik (France)
L. Fåhraeus (Sweden)
H. L. Judd (USA)
L. Schenkel (Switzerland)
J. W. W. Studd (UK)
M. I. Whitehead (UK)

INTRODUCTION

During the last five years much attention has been focused upon the hazards of oestrogens on the endometrium and other potentially adverse effects have been less comprehensively investigated. Although oestrogen therapy has been associated with hypertension (Crane *et al.*, 1971) and with cardiovascular and gall-bladder disease (Gow and MacGillivray, 1971; Boston Collaborative Drug Surveillance Program, 1972; Rosenberg *et al.*, 1976; Stein *et al.*, 1976), the validity of certain of the reports remains disputed as other data indicate a reduction in risk of death from cardiovascular disease with long-term oestrogen exposure (Ross *et al.*, 1981). Adverse changes in fibrinolytic/coagulation mechanisms have been observed during oestrogen therapy (Åstedt, 1971; Coope *et al.*, 1975), but it is not clear if these side effects are caused by all oestrogens, or if they are dose-dependent. Meaningful, comparative data on the biological effects and relative potencies of different oestrogens are incomplete and this is partially due to a lack of pertinent studies and also to a failure to appreciate that different end-organs and physiological systems exhibit quite dissimilar sensitivities to exogenous oestrogens. For example, Geola *et al.*, (1980) have reported that in post-menopausal women conjugated equine oestrogens 1.25 mg/day exhibited supra-physiological effects on the hepatic synthesis of renin substrate, physio-logical actions on the vaginal epithelium, and sub-physiological activity in terms of suppression of gonadotrophin levels. Thus, the biological effects of oestrogens can vary, being dependent upon the system under investigation, and truly physiological replacement therapy for every responsive end-organ may not be attainable with one oestrogen dose. Therefore, comparative studies on the potencies of different oestrogens must monitor changes within the same physiological system.

Much of the earlier work which compared oestrogenic potencies used suppression of circulating gonadotrophin concentrations or changes in total lipid levels as the oestrogen-responsive indices (Bolton, 1976). However, it has recently been suggested that changes in the rates of synthesis of certain hepatically-derived proteins and globulins, such as renin substrate, and cortisol (CBG) and sex hormone binding globulin (SHBG:TeBG) are more sensitive markers of oestrogen stimulation (Geola *et al.*, 1980). Marked alterations in hepatic metabolism due to oestrogens may have important clinical implications as the liver partially or wholly synthesizes renin substrate, high density lipoprotein (HDL) and low-density lipoprotein (LDL) moieties, and anti-thrombin III which, respectively, may influence the risk of hypertension, hyper-lipidaemia and arterial thromboembolic disease, and hypercoagulability and venous thromboembolic phenomena. Increases in the circulating levels of renin substrate have been proposed as a possible basis for the elevation in blood pressure observed with oestrogen therapy through increased generation of angiotensin (Laragh *et al.*, 1967) and induction of abnormal and more active variants of this protein (Eggena *et al.*, 1978). Decreased HDL-cholesterol concentrations and a low HDL:LDL ratio are associated with an increased incidence of cerebrovascular accident and myocardial infarction (Gordon *et al.*, 1977; Yaari *et al.*, 1981) and the effects of synthetic and natural oestrogens on these lipo-protein moieties appear dissimilar (Wallentin and Larsson-Cohn, 1977). Anti-thrombin III is currently believed to be of special importance in preventing intravascular thrombosis. An increased incidence of throm-botic episodes is associated with inherited anti-thrombin III deficiency states (van der Meer *et al.*, 1973; Mackie *et al.*, 1978), and the predis-position towards thrombosis occurring during oral contraceptive therapy has been related to synthetic oestrogens depressing anti-thrombin III levels (von Kaulla and von Kaulla, 1970; Sager *et al.*, 1976).

It has also been proposed that these hepato-cellular effects are related not only to the type of oestrogen but also to the route of administration. Oral therapy may result in a large, unphysiological 'bolus' of oestrogen being delivered directly into hepatic tissue via the portal circulation. Conversely, parenteral routes of administration, such as subcutaneous implantation and percutaneous absorption, deliver the oestrogen into the systemic circulation and therefore may cause less marked changes in hepatic biosynthesis because the portal system is by-passed.

The principal questions discussed in this workshop were, firstly, what are the relative potencies of the currently available oral oestrogens, and, secondly, does parenteral administration cause less profound hepato-cellular effects than the oral route? The data which helped resolve these issues also provided information on the relative sensitivities of different end-organs and physiological systems in the post-menopausal woman to exogenous oestrogens, differences in biological effects between natural and synthetic oestrogens, and the pharmaco-dynamics of oestradiol and oestrone after parenteral administration.

The conclusions and recommendations of the two previous meetings of the International Menopause Society (van Keep *et al.*, 1976, 1979) were agreed by consensus, but at this symposium the personal opinions of the moderator and secretary were sought and are as stated below. To allow the individual reader to draw his/her own conclusions, much of the original data presented are reproduced in detail.

RELATIVE POTENCIES OF ORAL OESTROGENS

This aspect was discussed by *Brenner* and by *Judd*. Both presented data (Figures 1 and 2) on changes in the circulating levels or binding capacity

(BC) of follicle stimulating hormone (FSH) and the liver-derived proteins and globulins, renin substrate, cortisol binding globulin (CBG) and sex hormone binding globulin (SHBG) following administration to post-menopausal women either of different dosages of the same oestrogen, or of various natural and synthetic oestrogens. One of the principal aims of *Judd*'s study was to ascertain the dosages of conjugated equine oestrogens and ethinyloestradiol which provided *physiological* replacement. Four dosages of conjugated equine oestrogens (0.15, 0.30, 0.625 and 1.25 mg/day) and of ethinyloestradiol (5, 10, 20 and 50 μg/day) were evaluated and comparative data were obtained from pre-menopausal women and an untreated, control group of post-menopausal subjects. Part of this study has been published elsewhere (Geola *et al.*, 1980) and only the conjugated equine oestrogen data are presented here. *Brenner*'s group was more concerned with establishing potency equivalents between the currently available natural and synthetic oestrogens and thus monitored the effects of four dosages of conjugated equine oestrogens, five dosages of piperazine oestrone sulphate, and two dosages of micronized oestradiol, ethinyloestradiol, and diethylstilbestrol (Figure 2).

Comparisons between the two sets of data are not intended and would be inappropriate given the somewhat different clinical and laboratory methodology and expression of results. A significant depression of FSH levels was observed with dosages of conjugated equine oestrogens exceeding 0.3 mg/day (Figure 1) although values within the pre-menopausal range were not achieved by the highest dose of 1.25 mg/day. Dose-dependant suppression of FSH was also present with all dosages of piperazine oestrone sulphate, and with both dosages of micronized oestradiol and diethylstilbestrol (Figure 2).

The baseline values of renin substrate, CBG and SHBG in the untreated post-menopausal women were within the pre-menopausal range, and dose-dependant elevations were observed during conjugated equine oestrogen therapy (Figure 1). The lowest dosages which achieved significant increases above the baseline were 0.15 mg/day for SHBG, 0.3 mg/day for renin substrate, and 0.625 mg/day for CBG (Figure 1). *Judd* also reported that the smallest dose of ethinyloestradiol, 5 μg/day, significantly increased renin substrate and SHBG concentrations, and that 10 μg/day elevated CBG to levels greater than the pre-menopausal range (data not shown). Similar dose-response relationships were present with the other oestrogen preparations studied by *Brenner*'s group (Figure 2) with the exception of changes in CBG during treatment with micronized oestradiol.

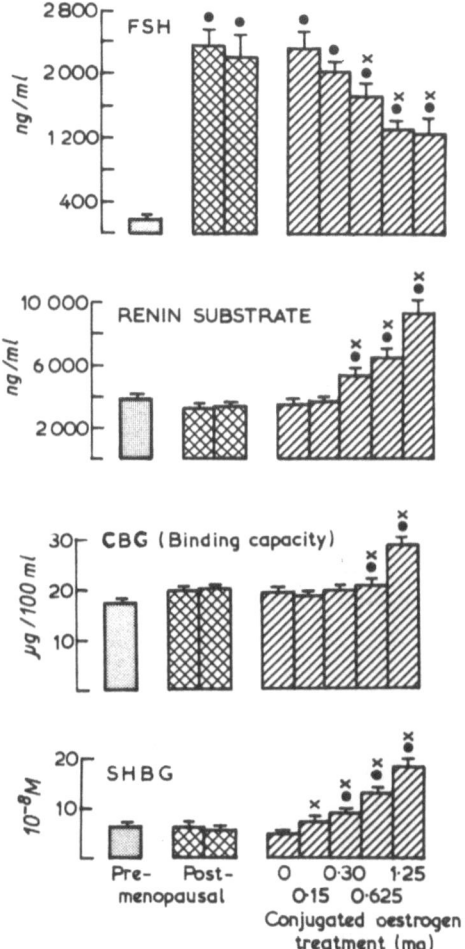

Figure 1 Mean (±SE) serum concentrations of FSH, renin substrate, SHBG, and the serum binding capacity of CBG in pre-menopausal women, untreated post-menopausal subjects on two occasions, and oestrogen-exposed post-menopausal women before (0) and then after the stated daily doses of conjugated equine oestrogens.

FSH = Follicle stimulating hormone; CBG = Cortisol binding globulin; SHBG = Sex hormone binding globulin.

Statistical differences between groups were determined by Student's two-tailed t test and the difference in values of subjects studied repetitively was evaluated by Student's paired t test.

• = Significant difference ($p<0.01$) from the pre-menopausal group.

× = Significant difference ($p<0.05$) from baseline post-menopausal values.

(Adapted from Geola *et al.*, 1980, *J. Clin. Endocrinol. Metab.*, **51**, 620, and reproduced with permission of the authors and of the editor)

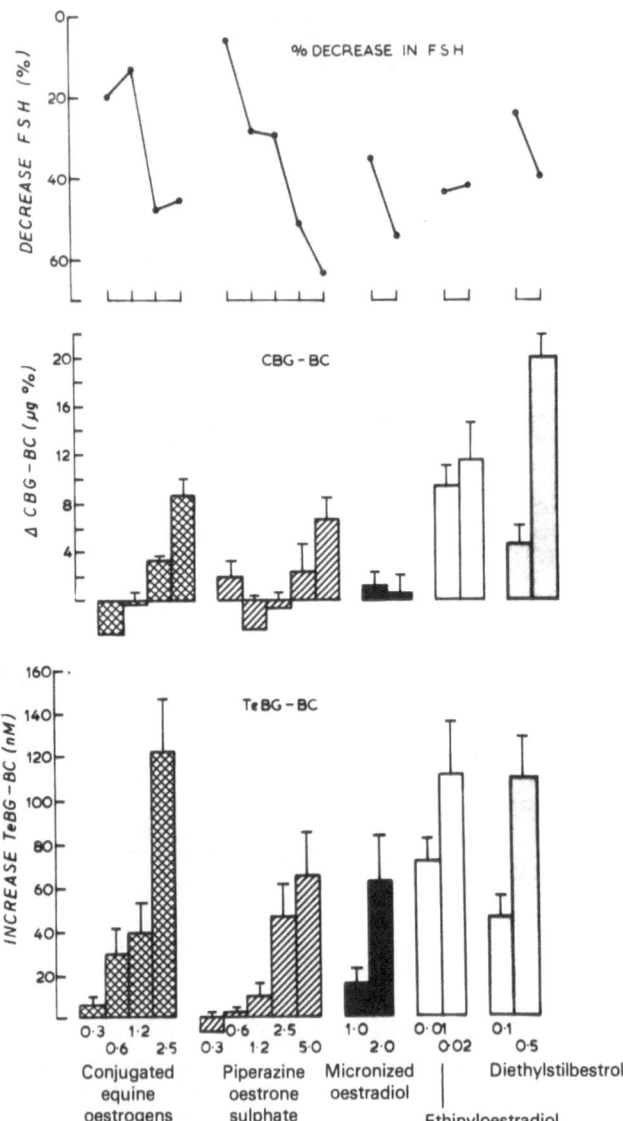

Figure 2 Percentage decrease in the circulating levels of FSH and changes in the serum CBG-BC and TeBG-BC in post-menopausal women receiving varying doses of natural and synthetic oestrogens.

FSH = Follicle stimulating hormone; CBG-BC = Binding capacity of cortisol binding globulin; TeBG-BC = Binding capacity of sex hormone binding globulin.

Dosages are in mg/day.

(Reproduced by kind permission of P. F. Brenner, C. A. Mashchak, R. A. Lobo, D.-K. Ryoko, D. Eggena, R. M. Nakamura and D. R. Mishell, Jr)

Table 1 Relative potencies of natural and synthetic oestrogens on four physiological systems in post-menopausal women. The results are expressed in mg-equivalents of piperazine oestrone sulphate

Oestrogen preparation	Serum FSH	Serum CBG-BC	Serum SHBG-BC	Serum renin substrate
Piperazine oestrone sulphate	1.0	1.0	1.0	1.0
Micronized oestradiol	1.3	1.9	1.0	0.7
Conjugated equine oestrogens	1.4	2.5	3.2	3.5
Diethylstilbestrol	3.8	70	28	13
Ethinyloestradiol	80–200*	1000*	614	232

*Extrapolation of results in the absence of parallelism.
FSH = Follicle stimulating hormone; CBG-BC = Binding capacity of cortisol binding globulin; SHBG-BC = Binding capacity of sex hormone binding globulin.
(Reproduced by kind permission of P.F. Brenner, C.A. Mashchak, R.A. Lobo, D.-K. Ryoko, D. Eggena, R.M. Nakamura and D.R. Mishell, Jr.)

The potencies of the various natural and synthetic oestrogen preparations studied by *Brenner*'s group were determined by parallel, live analyses and are shown in Table 1, expressed in mg-equivalents of piperazine oestrone sulphate. The hepatic responses of renin substrate were the most sensitive and those of CBG-BC the least. On a weight-for-weight basis, piperazine oestrone sulphate and micronized oestradiol exhibited similar potencies in each of the four systems studied, and their effects on hepatic synthesis were the least exaggerated relative to suppression of FSH levels. Conjugated equine oestrogens produced similar responses to piperazine oestrone sulphate and micronized oestradiol in suppression of FSH concentrations but were two to three times more potent in all three hepatic systems. The two synthetic oestrogens, ethinyloestradiol and diethylstilbestrol, produced more marked responses in every system and, importantly, their hepatic potency was between four and eighteen-fold in excess of that estimated from their suppression of FSH.

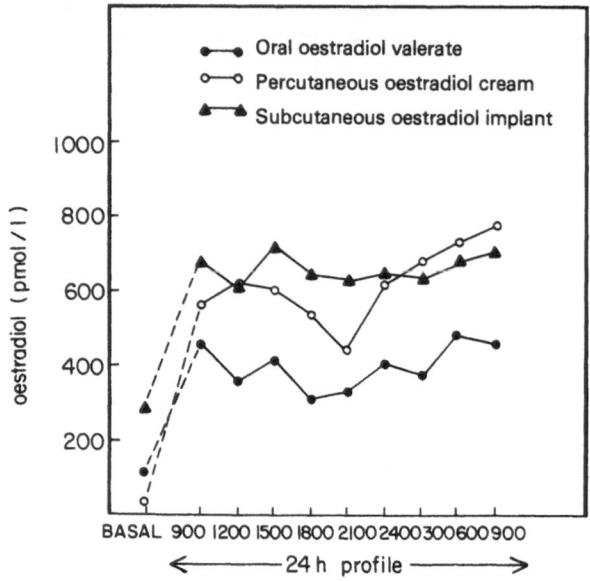

Figure 3 Mean plasma oestradiol levels in post-menopausal women before and then during therapy with orally, percutaneously, and subcutaneously administered oestradiol preparations. For details of dosages see text.
(Reproduced by kind permission of P. T. Townsend, G. Dyer, O. Young and M. I. Whitehead)

OESTROGEN EFFECTS AFTER DIFFERENT ROUTES OF ADMINISTRATION

Plasma levels of oestrone and oestradiol following administration of oral oestradiol valerate 2 mg/day, percutaneous oestradiol cream 5 g/day (i.e., a dose of 3 mg oestradiol), and subcutaneous oestradiol implants 50 mg were presented by *Whitehead* and are shown in Figures 3 and 4. All patients (at least five per treatment group) received therapy for between six and ten weeks before the 24 hour profiles were performed. Oral oestradiol valerate was associated with the smallest rise in plasma oestradiol levels (Figure 3) but with the most marked increases in oestrone concentrations (Figure 4). Tablets were ingested at 21.00 hours and a surge in oestrone values was observed shortly thereafter and maintained until 06.00 hours the following morning. Percutaneous and

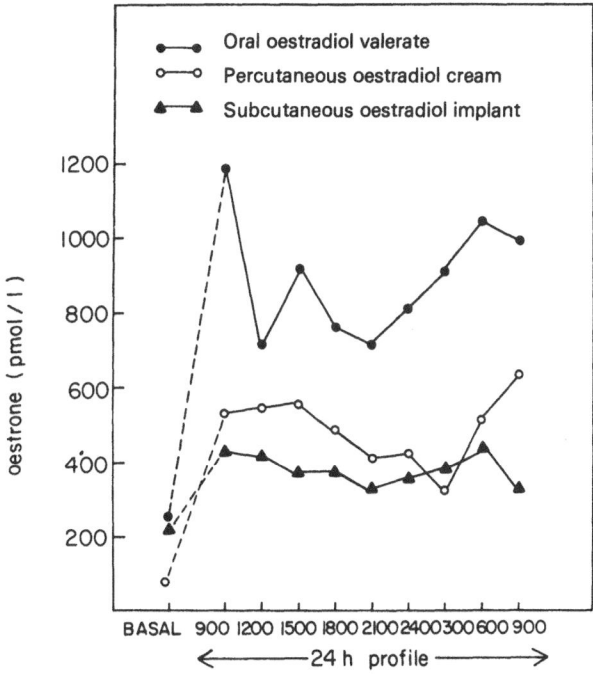

Figure 4 Mean plasma oestrone levels in post-menopausal women before and then during therapy with orally, percutaneously, and subcutaneously administered oestradiol preparations. For details of dosages see text.
(Reproduced by kind permission of P. T. Townsend, G. Dyer, O. Young and M. I. Whitehead)

subcutaneous oestradiol produced comparable oestrone and oestradiol levels well within the pre-menopausal proliferative phase range and there was little, if any, diurnal variation in the levels of either oestrogens with implant therapy. However, percutaneous administration at 21.00 hours was followed, within 3 hours, by an increase in plasma oestradiol concentrations which was sustained for at least 12 hours. The rise in oestrone values was slower, commencing three to six hours after application of the cream, and less marked. Identical patterns have been reported previously (Whitehead *et al.*, 1980).

Schenkel presented preliminary, pharmaco-dynamic data using a transdermal therapeutic system (TTS). This system consists of two membranes approximately 3 cm in diameter, enclosing a reservoir of oestradiol. The lower membrane is covered by adhesive and is permeable to the steroid, being applied to the skin for periods of between 24 and 72 hours. The upper membrane is occlusive and impermeable. Two dosage

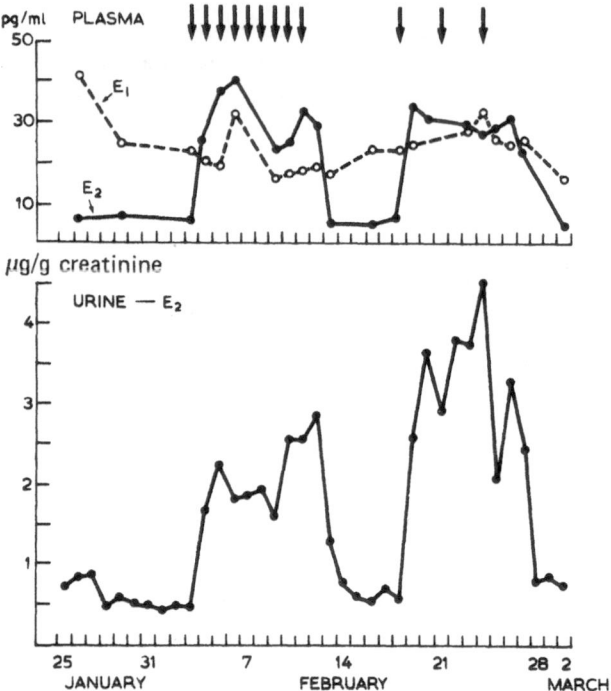

Figure 5 Plasma oestradiol (E_2) and oestrone (E_1) levels and urinary oestradiol concentrations in a post-menopausal woman before, during, and after application of two transdermal therapeutic systems (TTS). Arrows indicate days of TTS application. (Reproduced by kind permission of L. Schenkel)

systems have been developed, one to deliver 15 to 30 µg of oestradiol/day and the other 30 to 60 µg/day. Changes in plasma oestrone and oestradiol and urinary oestrogen concentrations during application of two TTS each day to a post-menopausal woman are shown in Figure 5. In the first study, between February 3rd and 11th, the two TTS were renewed daily for nine consecutive days whereas in the second investigation, between February 18th and 27th, they were renewed every 72 hours. The increase in plasma oestradiol concentrations was more marked than for oestrone and corresponding increases in the urinary oestrogen excretion were observed.

Data comparing the effects of oral and percutaneously administered oestrogens on suppression of gonadotrophin levels and induction of hepatic synthesis were presented by *Fåhraeus* and by *Elkik*. In a six-month study, 38 symptomatic, post-menopausal women were randomly allocated by *Fåhraeus*'s group to treatment with percutaneous oestradiol

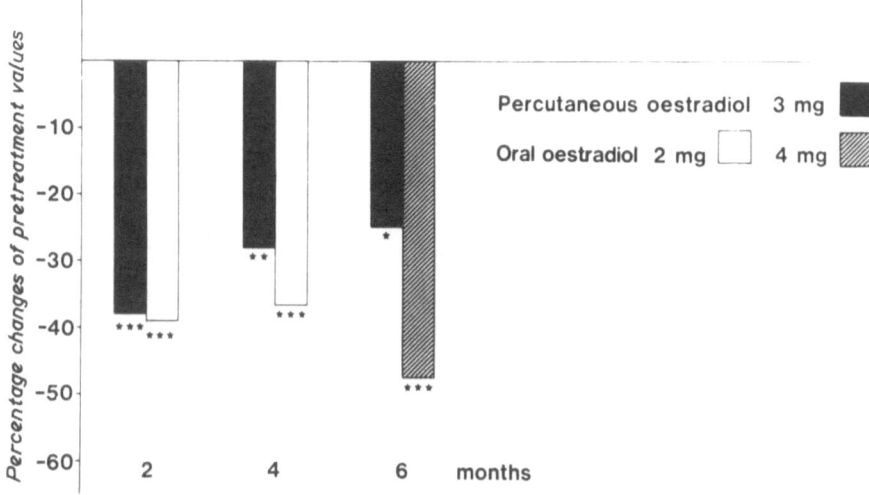

Figure 6 Percentage changes in FSH levels in post-menopausal women at two-monthly intervals following administration of percutaneous and of oral oestradiol preparations. For details of dosages see text.
Statistical comparisons of values before and during treatment by Student's paired t test.
  *$p < 0.05$
  **$p < 0.01$
  ***$p < 0.001$
(Reproduced by kind permission of L. Fåhraeus, L. Wallentin and U. Larsson-Cohn)

cream 5 g/day (i.e., a dose of 3 mg oestradiol) or oral micronized oestradiol. The dosage of the oral preparation was 2 mg/day for 4 months and then 4 mg/day. Changes in FSH and HDL-cholesterol levels are illustrated in Figures 6 and 7. The FSH reductions observed with the two treatments were similar after two and four months of therapy but more pronounced at six months in the group in which the dosage of oral oestradiol had been increased to 4 mg/day (Figure 6). Oral oestradiol, 2 mg/day, was associated with a depression in total cholesterol, mainly due to a reduction in low density lipoprotein (data not shown), and with an increase in HDL-cholesterol (Figure 7) resulting primarily from rise in the HDL^2 fraction. An increase in dosage to 4 mg was associated with a rise in triglyceride levels. The only change observed during percutaneous oestradiol therapy was a decrease in low density lipoprotein after six months treatment (data not shown).

Elkik's group studied 18 post-menopausal subjects who received either oral conjugated equine oestrogens 1.25 mg/day (8 patients) or per-cutaneous oestradiol cream 5 g/day (i.e., a dose of 3 mg oestradiol)

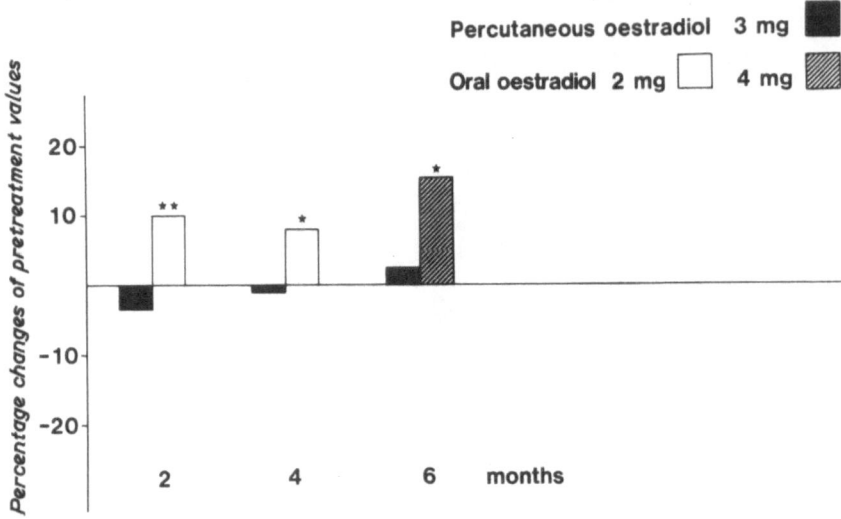

Figure 7 Percentage changes in HDL-cholesterol levels in post-menopausal women at two-monthly intervals following administration of percutaneous and of oral oestradiol preparations. For details of dosages see text.
Statistical comparisons and probabilities as in Figure 6.
(Reproduced by kind permission of L. Fåhraeus, L. Wallentin and U. Larsson-Cohn)

for 21 days. The changes in renin substrate, SHBG, and anti-thrombin III levels are shown in Table 2. Conjugated equine oestrogens significantly elevated renin substrate ($p < 0.01$) and SHBG ($p < 0.01$), and significantly reduced plasma anti-thrombin III levels ($p < 0.05$). Percutaneous oestradiol was without effect on renin substrate and anti-thrombin III, but increased SHBG ($p < 0.05$). However, the magnitude of the rise (19%) was markedly less than with conjugated equine oestrogens (150%).

Another index of liver/oestrogen interaction was presented by *White-head* whose group measured peripheral oestrone-3-glucuronide concentrations. Glucuronidation of oestrogens occurs almost exclusively in hepatic tissue. No changes in the plasma levels were observed following oestradiol implant therapy (50 mg) or percutaneous administration of oestradiol (5 g/day cream; 3 mg oestradiol), but a two- to three-fold increase in oestrone-3-glucuronide values was present with oral oestradiol valerate 2 mg/day (Figure 8). The oral preparation was administered at 21.00 hours and the subsequent surge in oestrone-3-glucuronide levels, between 24.00 hours and 09.00 hours the following morning, corresponded with an almost identical change in plasma oestrone concentrations (cf. Figure 4).

Table 2   Mean (±SE) plasma levels of renin substrate, anti-thrombin III, and sex hormone binding globulin in post-menopausal women before and after therapy with conjugated equine oestrogens (1.25 mg/day) and percutaneous oestradiol (3 mg/day)

		Before treatment	After treatment	% Variation	p
Renin substrate (ng Angiotensin I ml^{-1} h^{-1})	Conjugated oestrogens	0.94±0.10	2.49±0.90	+ 180±35.3	<0.01
	Percutaneous oestradiol	1.00±0.07	0.94±0.10	+ 6.0±3.5	N.S.
Anti-thrombin III (ng/ml)	Conjugated oestrogens	34.73±1.26	30.33±1.12	− 12.0±3.8	<0.05
	Percutaneous oestradiol	31.56±1.65	32.06±1.37	+ 1.5±0.4	N.S.
Sex hormone binding capacity (nmol/l)	Conjugated oestrogens	78.63±14.70	170.84±18.34	+ 150.0±41.0	<0.01
	Percutaneous oestradiol	70.20±8.01	82.32±9.04	+ 18.6±16.0	<0.05

Statistical comparisons of values before and after treatment by Wilcoxon's test.
N.S. = not significant.
(Reproduced by kind permission of F. Elkik, A. Gompel and P. Mauvais-Jarvis)

Studd presented data on the beneficial effects of implant therapy on a variety of climacteric and post-menopausal complaints including vasomotor instability, insomnia, dyspareunia, and minor degrees of psychological retardation. Particular emphasis was placed upon the value of implant therapy in the management of psycho-sexual problems such as loss of libido and anorgasmia. In a prospective study post-menopausal women were allocated to implant therapy with either oestradiol alone (30 or 50 mg) or oestradiol plus testosterone (100 mg). The control group underwent the usual preparations for implantation, including skin incision, but no implant was inserted. Assessment was performed at monthly intervals by a psycho-sexual counsellor unaware of the treatment regimen. The frequency of orgasm was unchanged in the controls and in the group receiving oestradiol alone, but markedly increased in the group receiving combined oestradiol and testosterone therapy. Earlier observations (Studd, 1979) were thus confirmed.

Finally, *Whitehead* presented data on endometrial stimulation with oral oestradiol valerate (2 mg/day) percutaneous oestradiol (5 g/day

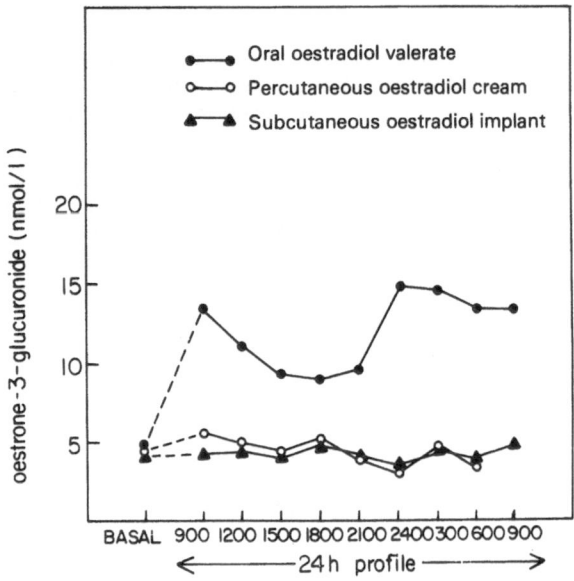

Figure 8 Mean plasma oestrone-3-glucuronide levels in post-menopausal women before and then during therapy with orally, percutaneously, and subcutaneously administered oestradiol preparations. For details of dosages see text.
(Reproduced by kind permission of G. Dyer, O. Young, P. Townsend and M. I. Whitehead)

cream; 3 mg oestradiol) and subcutaneous oestradiol implants (50 mg). Oestrogenic potency was assessed by measurements of soluble progesterone (RPC) and nuclear oestradiol receptor (REN), and comparative data from post-menopausal women receiving oral conjugated equine oestrogens, 1.25 mg/day, and from pre-menopausal proliferative and luteal phase endometria were included for comparison (Figure 9). All preparations gave RPC values at least equal to pre-menopausal, proliferative phase samples, and oestradiol implants induced hyperphysiological levels (Student's t test: $p < 0.05$). Oral oestradiol valerate and oestradiol implants gave REN values within the proliferative phase range and although the mean level with percutaneous oestradiol was lower the difference was not significant ($p > 0.1$).

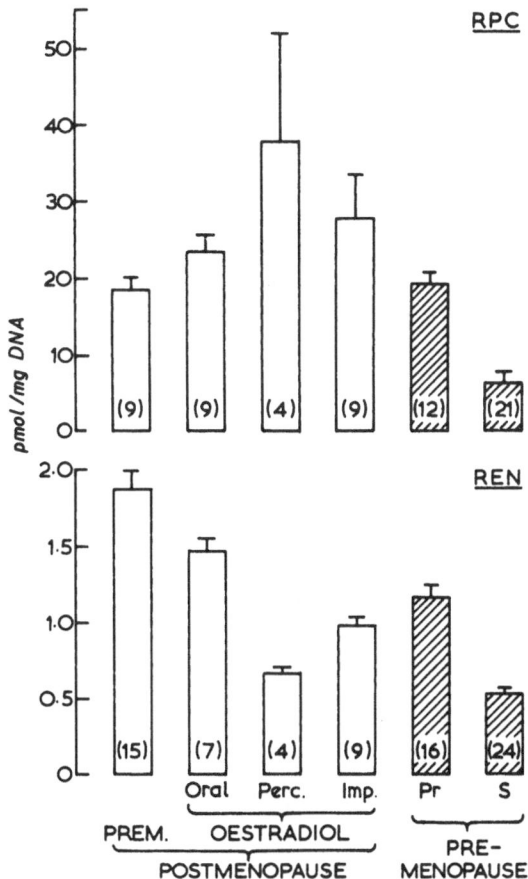

Figure 9 Soluble progesterone (RPC) and nuclear oestradiol receptor (REN) content of endometria from post-menopausal women receiving oral, percutaneous and subcutaneous oestradiol preparations, and oral conjugated equine oestrogens. Comparative data from pre-menopausal proliferative (Pr) and secretory (S) phase samples are included for comparison. For details of dosages see text.
Results are expressed as mean ± SE (number of observations).
(Reproduced by kind permission of M. I. Whitehead, P. T. Townsend, N. C. Siddle, G. Lane and R. J. B. King)

DISCUSSION

It is clear from the data presented here that the various oral oestrogen preparations currently available influence and alter different physiological systems within the post-menopausal woman in quite dissimilar ways. The 'natural' oestrogens, piperazine oestrone sulphate, micronized oestradiol, and conjugated equine oestrogens, are almost equipotent in terms of suppression of FSH, and piperazine oestrone sulphate and micronized oestradiol cause similar changes in hepatic synthesis. However, the hepato-cellular effects of conjugated equine oestrogens are two to three times more marked (Figure 2, Table 1). Expressed slightly differently, comparable dosages of these three natural oestrogens in terms of stimulation of hepatic metabolism are piperazine oestrone sulphate 1.25 mg, micronized oestradiol 1 mg, and conjugated equine oestrogens 0.3 mg. As the oestrone component of conjugated equine oestrogens gives similar plasma oestrone and oestradiol concentrations to those observed with piperazine oestrone sulphate and oral oestradiol (Whitehead, 1978), the data suggest that the equine components of conjugated oestrogens, equilin and 17α dihydroequilin, possess intrinsic activity.

The synthetic oestrogens, ethinyloestradiol and diethylstilbestrol are, on a weight-for-weight basis, markedly more potent than their natural counterparts in terms of FSH suppression (Table 1). These differences are exaggerated within the hepatic systems where the effects of ethinyloestradiol are 230–1000 and those of diethylstilbestrol 13–70 times more marked than those of piperazine oestrogen sulphate. After adjustment to give comparable FSH responses with the natural formulations, the hepato-cellular potencies of ethinyloestradiol and diethylstilbestrol were found to be 4–18 fold greater than those of the three natural preparations (Table 1).

The various liver systems do not respond equally to conjugated equine oestrogens. Significant increases above baseline were observed for SHBG with 0.15 mg/day, for renin substrate with 0.3 mg/day, and for CBG with 0.625 mg/day (Figure 1). Thus, not only do different physiological systems differ in their response to oestrogens but variations also occur within individual end-organs if they possess more than one function. Therefore assessment of absolute and relative potencies of oestrogens must be made on one specific function of an end-organ/physiological system since the effects on one activity may not reflect changes in another.

For reasons stated in the *Introduction*, changes in hepatic metabolism may have important clinical implications but not all of them should be regarded as being adverse. For example, increases in the circulating levels of SHBG and CBG have no known detrimental clinical effects and in theory may be beneficial. Increasing SHBG and CBG activity is likely to reduce excessive oestrogenic and progestational stimulation respectively as more of each steroid will be plasma-bound and therefore unavailable to responsive cells. Conversely, increases in renin substrate levels must be regarded as potentially adverse and the profound differences between natural and synthetic oestrogens on renin substrate induction reported here raise crucial questions regarding the most suitable form of treatment. The effects of 5 μg ethinyloestradiol approximated to those of 1.25 mg conjugated equine oestrogens (Table 1), but whilst there are good data showing beneficial effects of this dose of the natural oestrogen on climacteric symptomatology (Campbell and Whitehead, 1977) and bone status (Meema et al., 1975), there is no evidence that such low dosages of ethinyloestradiol are equally therapeutic. The usually prescribed dosages of ethinyloestradiol for relief of the symptoms of oestrogen deficiency range from 20 to 50 μg/day and totally unphysiological renin substrate concentrations can be predicted with these dosages since induction of the substrate is clearly dose-related (Figure 1). The implications for the post-menopausal woman are clear and to minimize possible undesirable changes in the renin–angiotensin system, and to keep them within the range observed with the natural oestrogens, the synthetic preparations must be prescribed at minute dosages, approximately 5 μg/day ethinyloestradiol and 0.1 mg/day diethylstilbestrol. It remains to be determined whether such small dosages are clinically effective.

It is also suggested that higher dosages of the natural oestrogen preparations be evaluated for their contraceptive efficacy, especially in the obese, older tobacco-user. Unlike that of synthetic oestrogens, the potency of the natural preparations in terms of reduction of FSH levels is relatively high when compared to their hepato-cellular effects (Table 1) and thus suppression of ovulation may be achieved with minimal disturbances in liver protein synthesis.

Possible explanations for the exaggerated effects of synthetic oestrogens on liver metabolism include a greater affinity for the oestrogen receptor, more available receptors due to higher oestrogenic stimulation, and prolonged nuclear occupation by the oestrogen–receptor complex. Too few data are available to confirm or refute the first suggestion and it is considered unlikely that more receptor is available since, as has been reported previously (King et al., 1979), responsive cells 'down-regulate' following prolonged oestrogen stimulation and receptor levels fall. The third explanation, that of prolonged nuclear occupation, has a basis in that synthetic oestrogens are not substrates for the enzyme oestradiol 17β dehydrogenase (King *et al.*, 1981a). In other oestrogen-dependant tissues this enzyme lowers oestrogen stimulation by converting the potent intra-cellular oestradiol into the less active oestrone (King *et al.*, 1981b). By virtue of their structure, the synthetic oestrogens may be more resistant than their natural counterparts to the processes of intra-cellular metabolism and degradation and thus their activity may be prolonged. Similar comments apply to the equine oestrogens, equilin and 17α-dihydroequilin, which comprise approximately 35% of conjugated oestrogens. Interestingly, the hepato-cellular potency of this preparation has been found to be between that of the entirely natural and the completely synthetic formulations.

In terms of minimizing changes in hepatic synthesis, the advantages of natural oestrogens appear to be further enhanced by delivery into the systemic as opposed to the portal circulation. Any study comparing the effects of conjugated equine oestrogens and oestradiol, however administered, on the circulating levels of renin substrate, anti-thrombin III, and SHBG, is likely to show more marked changes with the equine oestrogens, given their greater hepatic potency. However, the differences in the effects of orally administered conjugated equine oestrogens and percutaneous oestradiol reported here (Table 2) cannot, in our opinion, be explained solely by the greater hepato-cellular potency of the former. Conjugated equine oestrogens were found to induce significant increases in the levels of renin substrate and SHBG and reductions in anti-thrombin III values, whereas percutaneous oestradiol was without effect on renin substrate and anti-thrombin III and caused only a minimal elevation of SHBG concentrations, an increase of 19% as compared to the 150% rise observed with conjugated equine oestrogens. The clinical significance of changes in renin substrate and anti-thrombin III levels have been discussed previously and these data suggest that the thrombogenic and hypertensive potential of oestrogens may be reduced by parenteral administration. The increase in SHBG levels with percutaneous oestradiol indicates a hepato-cellular effect which for the reasons discussed above is unlikely to cause adverse clinical sequelae.

The relative lack of hepatic potency of percutaneous as opposed to orally administered oestradiol is apparent from a comparison of their effects on lipid metabolism. Percutaneous oestradiol, 3 mg/day for six months, caused no changes in HDL-cholesterol concentrations (Figure 7) and the only effect observed was of a reduction in the LDL concentrations at the last assessment. Conversely, an oral dosage of 2 mg/day significantly elevated HDL-cholesterol values (Figure 7) after two months of treatment, primarily because of a rise in the HDL^2 fraction, and was associated with the reduction in total cholesterol mainly due to a depression of LDL. Thus, both routes of administration increase the HDL:LDL ratio although the effects were more marked, and occurred earlier, with the oral preparation. These changes must be regarded as beneficial, as high HDL concentrations and high HDL:LDL ratios have been reported as affording protection against cardiovascular disease (Gordon et al., 1977; Yaari et al., 1981) and long-term post-menopausal oestrogen therapy has been associated with a reduction in death from myocardial infarction (Ross et al., 1981). Whether the greater spectrum of changes observed with oral oestradiol actually confers greater protection against cardiovascular disease than the more limited effects of percutaneous administration remains to be elucidated and must be carefully weighed against the other potentially adverse hypertensive and thrombogenic effects of oral therapy.

Increasing the oral dosage to 4 mg/day in the 5th and 6th months of therapy caused minimal further changes in HDL-cholesterol (Figure 7) but resulted in an increase in triglyceride levels which is regarded as undesirable. The effects on suppression of FSH were also marked with the higher dose (Figure 6).

At present, the two most widely used methods for administering oestrogens parenterally in Europe are percutaneously as a cream and subcutaneously by implantation. The methods give comparable circulating levels of oestradiol which are within the pre-menopausal proliferative phase range and higher than the oestrone concentrations (Figures 3 and 4). Thus, the plasma values are more physiological than those following oral administration of oestradiol which results in a greater rise of plasma oestrone than the parent steroid.

Comparisons of plasma oestrogen levels following administration of different preparations are often expressed as 'oestradiol:oestrone ratios' and may be based on the results from one or perhaps two plasma samples collected in a 24 hour period. Caution should be exercised in the interpretation of such data as the plasma profiles for oestradiol and oestrone presented here clearly demonstrate certain variations in the levels of both oestrogens which are dependant on the route of administration. The most constant values for oestradiol and oestrone during a 24 hour period were obtained with implant therapy. Percutaneous administration did not produce such constant values over a 24 hour period. The levels of both oestrogens started to decline 18 hours after administration of the cream and a further application produced a surge in both oestrogen concentrations, that of oestrone occurring 3–6 hours after oestradiol thus indicating that this is the time taken for conversion (Figures 3 and 4).

The most marked increase observed was that of plasma oestrone following oral administration of oestradiol valerate. The 'bolus' of steroid carried via the portal system into the liver must be considerable as it was sufficient to produce circulating oestrone concentrations that approached hyper-physiological levels for up to nine hours after oral intake (Figure 4). The delivery of this steroid mass into the liver every time a tablet is ingested has been likened to 'hitting the liver with a hammer every 24 hours' and may account, at least in part, for the exaggerated hepato-cellular effects of orally administered natural oestrogens as compared to their more peripheral activities such as suppression of FSH. Additionally, the close temporal relationship between the surge in oestrone concentrations with those of the major hepatic metabolite, oestrone-3-glucuronide (Figure 8), clearly indicates that steroid absorption is associated with significant liver synthesis and it is probable that much of the ingested oestrone is inactivated even before it reaches the systemic circulation. No such increases in plasma oestrone-3-glucuronide levels were observed with percutaneous and subcutaneous therapies, the values remaining within the pre-treatment range (Figure 8).

There are practical difficulties with implant therapy as administration is more complex and once inserted the implants are difficult to remove. The consensus opinion of the discussants with experience in this area was (a) that requests and indications for removal are rare providing proper patient evaluation and counselling have been undertaken and (b) that subcutaneous oestradiol and testosterone appear to be of particular benefit in the management of patients with loss of libido and anorgasmia. However, requests for implant therapy appear to be more common in patients unwilling to take tablets and failure to comply with instructions regarding oral progestin use can result in adverse changes in endometrial status (see below). All discussants who had evaluated percutaneous oestradiol reported high patient compliance with good relief of symptoms.

The rôle and clinical indications of the TTS (transdermal therapeutic system) warrant further evaluation. The use of adhesive membranes permeable to oestradiol to deliver a dose of steroid into the systemic circulation at a fixed rate represents a novel approach. Using this system plasma oestradiol concentrations have been found to be more elevated than those of oestrone (Figure 5); they were quickly increased following application to within the proliferative phase range, and rapidly returned to baseline after discontinuation of therapy. Corresponding changes in urinary oestrogen excretion were also observed.

Lastly, the levels of soluble progesterone and nuclear oestradiol receptor produced by oral, percutaneous and subcutaneous oestradiol should be noted (Figure 9). Most of the American epidemiological data associating post-menopausal oestrogen use with an increase in risk of endometrial cancer relate to conjugated equine oestrogens, and the endometrial effects of other oral and parenterally administered preparations are less well-documented. However, it is clear from the data presented here that orally administered oestradiol induces comparable receptor levels to conjugated equine oestrogens which are within the proliferative phase range and thus the similar rates of induction of hyperplasia by these treatments is not surprising (Whitehead 1978). Almost identical receptor levels have been presented elsewhere during therapy with the synthetic oestrogen, mestranol (King and Whitehead, 1980).

Percutaneous and subcutaneous oestradiol have been found to result in nuclear oestradiol receptor levels not significantly different from the proliferative phase range whilst hyper-physiological levels of progesterone receptor were induced by implant therapy. As oestradiol is the predominant intra-nuclear oestrogen in the endometrium of oestrogen-treated post-menopausal women (King et al., 1980; Whitehead et al., 1981a), therapies which selectively increase plasma oestradiol concentrations are likely to cause greater endometrial stimulation. Therefore, although routes of administration which by-pass the portal circulation may subsequently be shown to minimize the risk of hypertensive and thrombotic disease, their endometrial potency at these dosages is at least equal to, if not greater than, oral therapies. There is a corresponding need for adequate progestin to prevent excessive endometrial stimulation (Whitehead, 1978; Whitehead et al, 1981b) and such treatment has to be given orally. As discussed previously, patients receiving implant therapy are often unwilling to take tablets and non-compliance can result in heavy, unscheduled vaginal bleeding and is associated with a 56% incidence of endometrial hyperplasia (Studd et al., 1980). It remains to be determined whether progestins can also be successfully administered parenterally.

References

Åstedt, B. (1971). Low fibrinolytic activity of veins during treatment with ethinyl oestradiol. Acta Obstet. Gynaecol. Scand., 50, 279

Bolton, C. H. (1976). The effects of ethinyl oestradiol and conjugated equine oestrogens on plasma lipids in oophorectomised women. In Campbell, S. (ed.) The Management of *the Menopause and Postmenopausal Years*, p. 185. (Lancaster: MTP Press)

Boston Collaborative Drug Surveillance Program (1972). Gall-bladder disease, venous disorders, breast tumors: relation to estrogens. *N. Engl. J. Med.*, **287**, 628

Campbell, S. and Whitehead, M. I. (1977). Oestrogen therapy and the menopausal syndrome. In Greenblatt, R. B. and Studd, J. W. W. (eds.) *Clinics in Obstetrics and Gynaecology. Vol. 4., no. 1, The Menopause*, p. 31. (Philadelphia and London: W. B. Saunders)

Coope, J., Thomson, J. M. and Poller, L. (1975). Effects of 'natural oestrogen' replacement therapy on menopausal symptoms and blood clotting. *Br. Med. J.*, **4**, 139

Crane. M. G., Harris, J. J. and Winsor, W. III (1971). Hypertension, oral contraception agents and conjugated oestrogens. *Ann. Intern. Med.*, **74**, 13

Eggena, P., Hidaka, H., Barrett, J. D. and Sambhi, M. P. (1978). Multiple forms of human plasma renin substrate. *J. Clin. Invest.*, **26**, 367

Geola, F. L., Frumar, A. M., Tataryn, I. V., Lu, K. H., Hershman, J. M., Eggena, P., Sambhi, M. P. and Judd, H. L. (1980). Biological effects of various doses of conjugated equine estrogens in postmenopausal women. *J. Clin. Endocrinol. Metab.*, **51**, 620

Gordon, T., Castelli, N. P., Hjortland, M. C., Kannel, W. B. and Dawber, T. R. (1977). High density lipoprotein as a protective factor against coronary artery disease. *Am. J. Med.*, **62**, 707

Gow, S. and MacGillivray, I. (1971). Metabolic, hormonal and vascular changes after synthetic oestrogen therapy in oophorectomised women. *Br. Med. J.*, **2**, 73

von Kaulla, E. and von Kaulla, K. N. (1970). Oral contraceptives and low anti-thrombin III activity. *Lancet*, **1**, 36

van Keep, P. A., Greenblatt, R. B. and Albeaux-Fernet, M. (eds.) (1976). *Consensus on Menopause Research* (Lancaster: MTP Press)

van Keep, P. A., Serr, D. M. and Greenblatt, R. B. (eds.) (1979). *Female and Male Climacteric* (Lancaster: MTP Press)

King, R. J. B., Dyer, G., Collins, W. P. and Whitehead, M. I. (1980). Intracellular estradiol, estrone and estrogen receptor levels in endometria from postmenopausal women receiving estrogens and progestins. *J. Steroid Biochem.*, **13**, 377

King, R. J. B., Townsend, P. T., Siddle, N. C. and Whitehead, M. I. (1981a). Mechanisms of progestin action on human endometrium. In Witliff, J. and Dapunt, O. (eds.) *Hormone Cell Interactions in Reproductive Tissues* (New York: Masson)

King, R. J. B., Townsend, P. T. and Whitehead, M. I. (1981b). The role of oestradiol dehydrogenase in mediating progestin effects on endometrium from postmenopausal women receiving oestrogens and progestins. *J. Steroid Biochem.*, **14**, 235

King, R. J. B. and Whitehead, M. I. (1980). Application of steroid receptor analyses to clinical and biological investigations of the postmenopausal endometrium. In Bresciani, S. (ed.) *Perspectives in Steroid Receptor Research*, pp. 259–271 (New York: Raven Press)

King, R. J. B., Whitehead, M. I., Campbell, S. and Minardi, J. (1979). Effect of oestrogen and progestin treatments on endometria from postmenopausal women. *Cancer Res.*, **39**, 1094

Laragh, J. H., Sealey, J. E., Ledingham, J. G. and Newton, M. A. (1967). Oral contraceptives; renin, aldosterone and high blood pressure. *J. Am. Med. Assoc.*, **201**, 918

Mackie, M., Bennett, B., Ogston, D. and Douglas, A. S. (1978). Familial thrombosis: inherited deficiency of anti-thrombin III. *Br. Med. J.*, **1**, 136

Meema, S., Bunker, M. L. and Meema, H. E. (1975). Preventive effect of oestrogen on postmenopausal bone loss. *Arch. Intern. Med.*, **135**, 1436

van der Meer, J., Stoepman van Dalen, E. A. and Jensen, J. M. S. (1973). Anti-thrombin III deficiency in a Dutch family. *J. Clin. Pathol.*, **26**, 532

Rosenberg, L., Armstrong, B., Phil, D. and Jick, H. (1976). Myocardial infarction and estrogen therapy in postmenopausal women. *N. Engl. J. Med.*, **294**, 1256

Ross, R. K., Paganini-Hill, A., Mack, T. M., Arthur, M. and Henderson, B. E. (1981). Menopausal oestrogen therapy and protection from death from ischaemic heart disease. *Lancet*, **1**, 858

Sager, S., Stamatakis, J. D., Thomas, D. P. and Kakkar, V. V. (1976). Oral contraceptives, anti-thrombin III activity and post-operative deep vein thrombosis. *Lancet*, **1**, 509

Stein, W. P., Brown, B. W., Haskell, W. L., Farquhar, T. W., Wherland, C. L. and Wood, P. D. S. (1976). Cardiovascular risk and use of estrogens or estrogen/ progestagen combinations. *J. Am. Med. Assoc.*, **235**, 811

Studd, J. W. W. (1979). The climacteric syndrome. In van Keep, P. A., Serr, D. M. and Greenblatt, R. B. (eds.) *Female and Male Climacteric* (Lancaster: MTP Press)

Studd, J. W. W., Thom, M. H., Paterson, M. E. L. and Wade-Evans, T. (1980). The prevention and treatment of endometrial pathology in postmenopausal women receiving exogenous oestrogens. In Pasetto, N., Paoletto, R. and Ambrus, J. L. (eds.) *Menopause and Postmenopause*, p. 127 (Lancaster: MTP Press)

Wallentin, L. and Larsson-Cohn, U. (1977). Postmenopausal oestrogen replacement and lipids. *Lancet*, **2**, 1358

Whitehead, M. I. (1978). The effects of oestrogens and progestogens on the postmenopausal endometrium. *Maturitas*, **1**, 87

Whitehead, M. I., Lane, G., Dyer, G., Townsend, P. T., Collins, W. P. and King, R. J. B. (1981a). Oestradiol: the predominant intranuclear oestrogen in the endometrium of oestrogen treated postmenopausal women. *Br. J. Obstet. Gynaecol.*, **88**, 914

Whitehead, M. I., Townsend, P. T., Kitchin, Y., Dyer, G., Iqbal, M. J., Mansfield, M. D., Young, O. and Minardi, J. (1980). Plasma steroid and protein hormone profiles in post-menopausal women following topical application of oestradiol-17β. In Mauvais-Jarvis, P., Vickers, C. F. H. and Wepierre, J. (eds.) *Percutaneous Absorption of Steroids*, p. 231 (London: Academic Press)

Whitehead, M. I., Townsend, P. T., Pryse-Davies, J., Ryder, T. A. and King. R. J. B. (1981b). Effects of estrogens and progestins on the biochemistry and morphology of the postmenopausal endometrium. *N. Engl. J. Med.*, **305**, 1599

Yaari, S., Goldbourt, U., Even-Zohar, S. and Neufeld, H. N. (1981). Associations of serum high density lipoprotein and total cholesterol with cardiovascular and cancer mortality in a 7-year prospective study of 10,000 men. *Lancet*, **1**, 1011

Workshop 13

Progestins in the peri-menopause

Moderator: **M. Notelovitz** (USA)

Speakers: **R. D. Gambrell** (USA)
C. Lauritzen (West Germany)
M. Notelovitz (USA)
G. Samsioe (Sweden)
J. W. W. Studd (UK)
M. I. Whitehead (UK)

Since the first retrospective studies indicated in the mid-1970s that the risk of endometrial cancer from post-menopausal oestrogen use was increased 4.6 to 8-fold, a 10–14-day course of progestogens has been advocated for routine usage with oestrogen replacement therapy (ERT) (Gambrell, 1978). Progestogens have, however, been shown to have a potentially adverse effect on both carbohydrate and lipid metabolism. The possibility therefore exists that the prevention of one disease (endometrial cancer) might provoke another (atherosclerosis), thereby negating the benefit of the currently advocated hormone replacement regime. This workshop set out to redefine the efficacy and need for combined oestrogen/progestogen therapy, and to evaluate the potential side-effects.

PREVENTION OF ENDOMETRIAL AND BREAST CANCER

Gambrell presented data to suggest that progestogens reduce the risk of endometrial cancer and may possibly afford some protection from breast cancer. His data were based on a total of 5563 post-menopausal women registered at Wilford Hall USAF Medical Center, and represent an accumulated total of 13 921 patient-years of observation. Between 1975 and 1979, 22 patients were found to have adenocarcinoma of the endometrium, an incidence of 158 per 100 000 women per year. The highest incidence was observed in the oestrogen-only users (434.4 per 100 000) and the lowest in the oestrogen/progestogen users (70.8 per 100 000). Not only did the oestrogen/progestogen users have a significantly lower incidence of endometrial cancer than the oestrogen users ($p < 0.001$), they also had a significantly lower incidence of this malignancy when compared to those who had never used hormones (242 per 100 000; $p < 0.05$).

Endometrial hyperplasia may be a pre-cancerous lesion in some women in that 30–48% of women with hyperplasia develop adenocarcinoma within 8–10 years. In the Wilford Hall studies, 325 post-menopausal women were treated with progestogens for 7–10 days each month and a curettage repeated after 3–6 months of therapy. Hyperplasia reversed to normal endometrium in 94.3%; in the 18 patients with persistent hyperplasia after progestogen therapy, 14 had been treated with progestogens for only 7 days of each month. This emphasizes the need to give a minimum of 10 days progestogen therapy each month in order to treat endometrial hyperplasia and prevent neoplasia.

Since the second-highest incidence of endometrial cancer was observed in the untreated group, i.e. in those never taking hormones, some method must be devised to identify women at greatest risk for endometrial cancer. Not all post-menopausal women need oestrogen therapy since many produce sufficient endogenous oestrogens to remain asymptomatic and prevent the associated metabolic changes of later life. It was recommended that all post-menopausal women with an intact uterus be given the *progestogen challenge test*. This includes both oestrogen-treated women and those patients with sufficient endogenous oestrogens. The progestogen should be continued for 10 days each month for as long as withdrawal bleeding results. It has been postulated that the use of the progestogen challenge test in this manner would prevent the majority of endometrial cancers (Gambrell *et al.*, 1980).

The causality between ERT and breast cancer was next discussed.

During a prospective study of hormone use at Wilford Hall, there were 24 599 patient years of observation. A total of 43 patients were found to have breast cancer during the 5 years of the study, an overall incidence of 174.8 per 100 000 women. The incidence of breast cancer was 137.3 per 100 000 in the oestrogen-only users and 95.6 per 100 000 in the oestrogen/progestogen users. Although the incidence of breast cancer in the oestrogen/progestogen users was lower than that of the oestrogen-only users, the difference was not statistically significant, but does indicate a trend ($p = 0.08$).

The prognosis of breast cancer was better in the hormone users than in the non-users in the Wilford Hall study. In those women who had never used hormones the mortality rate was 36.8% compared to 13.5% in the oestrogen-only users, and 14.3% in the oestrogen/progestogen users, which was statistically significant, $p < 0.01$. The improved prognosis in hormone-treated women most likely reflects an earlier diagnosis of breast cancer, although the possibility of a less virulent tumour must also be considered.

Scanning electronmicroscopy of the endometrium in post-menopausal women receiving oestrogens has confirmed both the stimulating effect of unopposed oestrogens and the inhibitory effect of added progestogens. *Studd* demonstrated examples of the normal scanning electronmicroscopic changes of the endometrium during the menstrual cycle. After 6 weeks of unopposed ERT, cystic hyperplasia may develop, with over a third of the surface cells being ciliated with long branched microvilli. In patients with adenomatous hyperplasia the cilia form a carpet over most of the surface. With atypical hyperplasia, areas of normal epithelium are interspersed with occasional large pleomorphic cells and some cilia formation. All cancer specimens are characterized by large pleomorphic cells with normal microvilli. Well-differentiated varieties may have occasional cilia. Treatment with prolonged courses of progestogen shows a reversal to normal with atrophic 'pill-like' flat regular cells devoid of cilia.

Studd also reported the results of a prospective study involving some 745 subjects. In this study high oestrogen-only usage was associated with abnormal endometrial histology in 14.8% of patients, low oestrogen treatment in 7% and oestrogen/progestogen treatment in 1.2%. The *duration* of progestogen therapy was directly related to the efficacy of its inhibitory function. The incidence of endometrial hyperplasia in women receiving oestrogen implants alone was 55.8%; when combined with a 5–7-day course of an oral progestogen (norethisterone 5 mg) the incidence fell to 8.3–12.5%; this was reduced further to 3% when progestogen treatment was extended to 10 days, and to 0% in patients receiving progestogens for more than 10 days/month (Paterson *et al.*, 1980).

METABOLIC SIDE-EFFECTS

Lipids and lipoproteins

Samsioe summarized his experience with progestogens and their effects on lipids and lipoproteins. The metabolic effects induced by a progestogen vary according to the degree of the progestogen's androgenicity, the route of administration, and, possibly, the duration of therapy. The presence of oestrogen is also important. Other factors need to be considered: most studies are based on a comparison of treated and non-treated populations; the indication for treatment may, in itself, play a major role in lipid metabolism; by alleviating symptoms (e.g. pain associated with endometriosis) the individual's increased physical activity can also influence and alter the metabolic outcome.

Samsioe drew attention to the results of a comparative study in oophorectomized women treated with norethisterone, with levonorgestrel, or with medroxyprogesterone acetate (MPA) (Silfverstolpe *et al.*, 1979). In this study norethisterone treatment resulted in a decrease of all the lipid components (triglycerides, cholesterol, phospholipids, LDL, HDL, VLDL, α-lipoproteins, lecithin, and fatty acid esters). Levonorgesterel caused a marked drop in HDL. The lipid composition of LDL was increased and that of VLDL decreased both by norethisterone and by levonorgestrel. Few changes were encountered after treatment with MPA. The fatty acid composition of the serum lecithin and cholesterol esters was unaffected by MPA. Levonorgestrel and, to a lesser extent, norethisterone produced a shift in palmitic and stearic acid indicating a reduction in the excretory function of the liver. This was confirmed by an increase in the BSP retention time. The effect of progestogens on lipids is altered when oestrogens are given simultaneously. This is probably mediated by the balance achieved between the hormonal effect (which depends on oestrogen receptors in the liver) and the drug effect (which is dependent on the liver's ability to conjugate and metabolize steroids) of sex steroid combinations. For example, progestogens counteract the hormonal effect of oestrogen, but act synergistically with oestrogens as far as conjugation and metabolism are concerned. Progestogens also decrease the stimulating effect of oestrogen on sex hormone binding globulin and alter the equilibrium and ratio between oestrone and oestradiol formation. In summary, progestogens have an anti-oestrogenic effect on lipids and lipoproteins, and tend to reduce HDL, VLDL, and to increase LDL. Although this effect decreases with the duration of hormone usage, age *per se* enhances the adverse effect of the combined sex steroids on HDL levels. Medroxyprogesterone and natural progesterone have less pronounced metabolic side-effects. The lipid and lipoprotein changes could be lessened if both oestrogens and progestogens could be given parenterally thereby avoiding the first liver passage.

Carbohydrate metabolism

Individuals with impaired glucose tolerance (2 h post-prandial blood glucose between 140 and 200 mg/dl) have an increased incidence of macroangiopathy. *Notelovitz* reviewed the evidence and suggested that both progesterone and progestogens have a potentially adverse affect on carbohydrate metabolism. For example, it is known that the control of diabetes is often impaired during the late luteal phase of the menstrual cycle and during menstruation, and that this is related to a significant decrease in insulin binding to circulating monocytes. Progesterone has also been shown to bind directly to the beta cells of the pancreas. By stimulating insulin release progesterone treatment results in the 'down regulation' of insulin receptors as observed in individuals with hyperinsulinaemia.

Clinical studies have shown that most of the progestogens used in practice, i.e. medroxyprogesterone acetate, megesterol acetate, and norgestrel, are associated with significant elevations of blood glucose and of plasma insulin (Spellacy *et al.*, 1976). Short-term therapy with progestogens (less than 6 months) is *not* associated with alterations in glucose or insulin metabolism. This is opposite to the effect that oestrogens have on glucose metabolism, and highlights the need to carefully assess the results of studies conducted over a relatively short period of time.

Experience with oral contraceptive usage has clearly shown that progestogens (either on their own or together with the synergistic action of oestrogens) create a state of absolute hyperinsulinaemia similar to that found in obese persons and maturity-onset diabetics – individuals prone to increased cardiovascular disease. Together with the suppressant effect that progestogens have on high-density lipoproteins, long-term oestrogen/progestogen therapy may, over a period of years, enhance an individual's liability to atherosclerosis. It must be emphasized that none of the above conclusions is based on the sex steroids currently recommended for ERT. However, in a recent study 3 months treatment with an oestrogen/progestogen combination (ethinyloestradiol megesterol acetate, or mestranol, or norethisterone) resulted in a 10–30% incidence of abnormal glucose tolerance compared to none in equally matched women treated with oestrogen alone. The potential for long-term oestrogen/progestogen treatment to result in subclinical abnormal glucose tolerance and hyperinsulinaemia clearly needs to be defined. There is a *theoretical* possibility that progestogen's ability to protect against oestrogen-induced endometrial hyperplasia and neoplasia, could be outweighed by an acceleration of atherogenesis.

Coagulation

The effect of combined oestrogen/progestogen hormone replacement therapy on coagulation has been evaluated by only a few investigators. In one study ethinyloestradiol 10 μg with megesterol acetate 1 mg for 5 days was studied and revealed no abnormalities in the dynamic functioning of coagulation, platelet activity or fibrinolysis. The mean anti-X_a activity was also unchanged. The doses used were lower than those usually recommended for replacement therapy. The same results were noted when natural oestrogens (conjugated oestrogen 0.625 and 1.25 mg; oestrone piperazine sulphate 1.5 and 3.0 mg) were combined with 5 days of norethisterone (2 and 5 mg), and when DL-norgestrel (0.5 mg) was added from day 12 to day 21 of cyclical oestradiol valerate. The parameters studied were: prothrombin time, partial thromboplastin time, fibrinogen levels, platelet aggregation, and factors X and VII. These studies were conducted over a relatively short period of time.

To evaluate the effect of combined oestrogen/progestogen therapy over an extended period (18 months) *Notelovitz* reported on the results of a prospective longitudinal study initiated at The Center for Climacteric Studies, University of Florida. Thirty-eight naturally menopausal women were studied. Eighteen subjects who elected not to receive ERT served as the control group. Their mean age was 53.4 years. The treatment group was randomly divided into those treated with 0.625 mg Premarin® (mean age, 49.6 years) and a second treatment group receiving 1.25 mg of Premarin® (mean age, 46.6 years). The two oestrogen-treated groups were also given 10 mg medroxyprogesterone acetate for 1 week during the third week of their 3-week cyclic oestrogen regime. Measurements of haematological parameters were made at the beginning of the study and at 6-month intervals thereafter for 18 months. The tests performed included: tests of dynamic function of coagulation (prothrombin time, activated partial thromboplastin time, thrombin time), tests indicative of intravascular coagulation (platelet count, fibrinogen antigen, fibrinogen activity, fibrin split products), tests indicative of natural anticoagulation (antithrombin III antigen and activity, α_1-antitrypsin antigen and α_2-macroglobulin antigen), and tests indicative of fibrinolysis (plasminogen antigen and activity). No adverse effects of treatment on coagulation and fibrinolysis could be demonstrated although the passage of time did induce changes in all groups suggestive of mild ongoing intravascular coagulation. This did not reach values compatible with a clinical effect and may have been compensated for by the increase in the α_1-antitrypsin antigen and the definite increase in fibrinolysis as reflected by increased plasminogen activity. This latter change was more pronounced in the hormone-treated groups.

As far as has been published to date, the addition of a progestogen does not affect the clotting mechanism adversely. In fact, if the experience of the progestogen-alone oral contraceptives and the above study are replicated, progestogens may actually improve the situation by enhancing fibrinolytic activity.

PHARMACOKINETICS AND TARGET TISSUE RESPONSE

Progestogens and progesterone are usually classified by structure and are divided into six major groups (Table 1). The majority of the progestogens are active orally. Bioavailability is improved if absorption is increased and metabolism delayed; this may be achieved by a variety of techniques which include decreasing particle size, imparting favourable substituted groups, and utilizing solvents with appropriate proton donation.

Until recently, natural progesterone was thought to be poorly absorbed and without an end-organ affect. *Whitehead* reported that plasma levels within the luteal phase range can be obtained 6 h after the oral administration of micronized progesterone (Whitehead *et al.*, 1980).

Since progestogens may have adverse metabolic and other side-effects, an attempt was made to determine the minimum dosage of

Table 1   Structural classification of progestins

Progestin	Derivatives
Progesterone	Progesterone
	Medroxyprogesterone acetate
	Megestrol acetate
Halogenated progesterone	Chlormadinone acetate
	Cyproterone
	Cyproterone acetate
Retro-progesterone	Dydrogesterone
19-norprogesterone	R-5020
	Gestonorone caproate
Testosterone	Dimethisterone
	Ethisterone
19-nortestosterone	Ethynodiol diacetate
	Lynestrenol
	Norethisterone (AC) (OEN)
	Norethynodrel
	Norgestrel

progestogens necessary to suppress endometrial proliferation effectively. The end-organ effects of the following were compared: four different dosages of norethisterone, two dosages of DL-norgestrel, and oral progesterone 300 mg daily, on the oestrogen-primed post-menopausal endometrium. Using sensitive biochemical indices of oestrogen and progesterone activities on endometrial samples, the data clearly showed that the currently recommended daily dosage of norethisterone, 10 mg daily and DL-norgestrel 500 µg daily, can be dramatically reduced to norethisterone 1 mg daily and DL-norgestrel 150 µg daily, without loss of effect. Electronmicroscopic studies confirmed that low dosages are just as effective as the higher daily dosages. Progesterone 300 mg daily exerted an effect on cell biochemistry similar to that of norethisterone 5 mg daily. Since progesterone may cause smaller changes in lipid and lipoprotein concentrations, further evaluation of natural progesterone treatment is warranted.

THE CLINICAL USE OF PROGESTOGENS

To place the clinical usage of progestogens into clear perspective, *Lauritzen* ended the series of formal presentations at this workshop by reporting on a recent survey of practice at the Women's Clinic, University of Ulm. In the clinic's pre-menopausal clientele of sex steroid treated patients, 31 % had received progestogens only, 51 % oestrogens and progestogens, 8% oestriol, 6% oestrogens and androgens, and 4% locally applied oestrogens. The main indications were hypermenorrhoea, menorrhagia, poly-oligomenorrhoea, mastopathy, premenstrual syndrome, therapeutic amenorrhoea. A small percentage of pre-climacteric women received oral contraceptives up to the age of 50 or more. During the menopause, oestrogen/progesterone treatment (12 days) was given to 50% of the cases up to the age of 55 years; 30% received oestriol, 10% oestrogens/androgens and 10% locally applied oestrogens. The main indication was typical climacteric symptomatology. In cases where only oestrogens were given, a progestogen withdrawal test was conducted once every 6 months. A retrospective evaluation of the cases at Ulm showed that the addition of a progestogen to the oestrogens does not cause additional risk. When oestrogens are contraindicated, progestogens alone are given.

The addition of a sufficient dose of a progestogen seems to decrease the likelihood of endometrial cancer. Glandular-cystic hyperplasia, atypical hyperplasia and Ca *in situ* can be reversed by progestogen therapy. Even endometrial, ovarian, and mammary cancers have been shown to regress.

DISCUSSION AND CONCLUSIONS

The value of progestogens in preventing oestrogen-stimulated hyperplasia was clearly endorsed. Emphasis was placed on the duration of treatment, a minimum of 10–14 days/month being required to ensure this effect. The latter was thought to be so effective that follow-up (annual or bi-annual) endometrial biopsy was no longer thought to be necessary, provided that a thorough examination of the endometrial cavity was made before the initiation of treatment. *Gambrell* highlighted the value of the 'progesterone challenge test'. The protective effect of progestogens on breast pathology was felt to be encouraging and it was hoped that once more cases had been studied its statistical benefit would be apparent.

The potential metabolic side-effects of progestogens have to be recognized and patients monitored accordingly by assessments of their blood lipids, lipoproteins, glucose, and regular checks on their blood pressure. However, it was felt that the benefit of progestogen therapy on the endometrium exceeded the 'potential' increased risk of cardiovascular disease.

Since the type and dosage of progestogen used will largely determine the clinical outcome, the restriction of progestogen usage to derivatives of progesterone and/or to the prescription of much lower doses of all progestogens should minimize unwanted side-effects without reducing the progestogens' endometrial inhibitory capacity.

References

Gambrell, R. D. (1978). The prevention of endometrial cancer in post-menopausal women with progestogens. *Maturitas,* **1**, 107

Gambrell, R. D., Massey, F. M., Castaneda, T. A., Ugenas, A. J., Ricci, C. A. and Wright, J. M. (1980). Use of the progestogen challenge test to reduce the risk of endometrial cancer. *Obstet. Gynecol.,* **55**, 732

Paterson, M. E. L., Wade-Evans, T., Sturdee, D., Thom, M. H. and Studd, J. W. W. (1980). Endometrial disease after treatment with oestrogens and progestogens in the climacteric. *Br. Med. J.,* **280**, 822

Silfverstolpe, G., Gustafson, A., Samsioe, G. and Svanborg, A. (1979). Lipid studies in oophorectomized women. Effects of three different progestogens. *Acta Obstet. Gynecol. Scand.,* **88**, (Suppl.), 89

Spellacy, W. N., Buhi, W. G. and Birk, S. A. (1976). The effects of orgestrel on carbohydrate and lipid metabolism over one year. *Am. J. Obstet. Gynecol.,* **125**, 984

Whitehead, M. I., Townsend, P. T., Gill, D. K., Collins, W. P. and Campbell, S. (1980). Absorption and metabolism of oral progesterone. *Br. Med. J.,* **280**, 825

Workshop 14

Epidemiologic aspects of the benefits and risks of oestrogen therapy

Moderator: **D. W. Cramer** (USA)

Speakers: **D. W. Cramer** (USA)
              I. Schiff (USA)

INTRODUCTION

This workshop attempted to summarize the epidemiologic evidence bearing on the proposed benefits and suspected risks of oestrogen therapy. We illustrated the sorts of data available, discussed their limitations and attempted to quantify their effects. The ultimate goal of this exercise was to permit some idea of the balance between risks and benefits of oestrogen therapy. From the outset, we concede that no simple equation can be derived to demonstrate a positive or negative balance sheet for oestrogen therapy. This is true because of gaps in our knowledge about the full effects of exogenous oestrogens, vagueness in the measures we use to value the risks and benefits, and widely different standards of practice which could affect risks and benefits.

NATURE OF EPIDEMIOLOGIC STUDIES

The epidemiologic evidence that can be brought to bear on this question includes simple descriptive studies, case–control and retrospective cohort studies and prospective clinical trials. By examining disease rates as they may vary by race, geography or time, correlations may be observed between those rates and the exposure which can be suggestive of a relationship. Case–control and retrospective cohort studies are the principal epidemiologic studies which attempt to quantify an association between exposure and illness and further qualify it as causal or non-causal. A well-designed prospective study is the best way to establish a relationship between exposure and outcome with any certainty but is rarely feasible to establish risks.

In case–control studies the starting population is defined by the presence or absence of the disease. Exposure in the diseased group is compared with exposure in the non-diseased controls. In retrospective cohort studies the starting population is defined by the presence or absence of an exposure which occurred in the past. The rate of disease that subsequently developed is determined in the exposed and non-exposed groups. The yield of both case–control and cohort studies is the relative risk which compares the exposed individual's risk relative to that of the non-exposed individual's risk.

A valid epidemiologic study is one that is free of three types of bias: observation or misclassification bias where subjects are misclassified with respect to exposure or disease, selection bias where cases and controls are selected in some way on a correlate of the exposure, or confounding due to factors such as age or race associated with both the exposure and illness. Alternatively associations which are strong, consistently found in different studies, show a dose response, and have biological credibility are unlikely to be spurious.

THE BENEFITS OF OESTROGEN THERAPY

The potential benefits of oestrogen therapy were considered under three headings: effects on the cardiovascular system, effects on bone, and effects on the central nervous system. Though recognized as a major benefit, relief of genital atrophy was not discussed in detail.

Descriptive studies of cardiovascular mortality in women show a steadily increasing rate with no sudden or dramatic upturn around the time of the menopause (Furman, 1971; Ryan, 1976). However, studies do indicate that women who have bilateral oophorectomy at an early age suffer an increased risk for cardiovascular death (Rosenberg *et al.*, 1976). It has not been established that replacement therapy can eliminate this risk. Case–control and cohort studies regarding oestrogens and cardiovascular disease have demonstrated neither increased nor decreased risk but have biases difficult to overcome in that women at risk for cardio-vascular disease may not be given oestrogens (Pfeffer *et al.*, 1978, Hammond *et al.*, 1979, Ross *et al.*, 1981). This contraindication arose from prospective studies that demonstrated high cardiovascular death rates in males with existing cardiovascular disease given high-dose oestrogen prophylaxis (Coronary Drug Project Research Group, 1970). But such studies are not generalizable to the woman without risk factors for cardiovascular disease placed on low-dose oestrogens. Indeed oestro-gens should be beneficial since they raise high-density lipoproteins (Bradley *et al.*, 1978). More studies are in order since even a small beneficial effect could have great impact.

In terms of osteoporosis, descriptive data reveal that fracture rates for post-menopausal women are many times that for men and are an important source of morbidity and mortality (Nordin, 1971; Gallagher and Nordin, 1974). In the case of osteoporosis we are in the unique position of having excellent prospective studies clearly demonstrating a beneficial effect of oestrogen (Lindsay *et al.*, 1976; Nachtigall *et al.*, 1979). It is just now that case–control studies are confirming a beneficial effect of oestrogens on bone fractures (Hutchinson *et al.*, 1979; Weiss *et al.*, 1980) and suggest that women who use oestrogens have one-third the risk for fractures as non-users. Thus there is little doubt that oestrogen together with dietary calcium can retard the bone loss that occurs with ageing, and maintain bone density above the fracture threshold. Pre-vention of osteoporosis is a major benefit of oestrogen that adds consider-able weight to the benefits side of the therapeutic equation.for replace-ment oestrogen.

Manifestations of oestrogen depletion on the central nervous system (CNS) may include flushes, insomnia, and mood changes. It is often difficult to quantify these variables but they clearly have substantial impact on the woman's quality of life. The only satisfactory way to establish the effect of oestrogen on such symptoms is through clinical trials using a placebo; and in such controlled studies, oestrogen has proven its efficacy in relieving hot flushes (Campbell, 1976; Coope, 1976; Schiff *et al.*, 1979). Since the CNS symptoms often occur in constellations, relief of hot flushes is often associated with improved sleep, memory, mood and other psychological variables (Campbell, 1976).

Finally, a brief word about therapeutic regimens for menopausal symptoms. Progesterone is effective against hot flushes (Schiff *et al.*,

1980a; Albrecht *et al.*, 1981) but does not have other major benefits and theoretically could have an adverse impact on cardiovascular disease. The use of vaginal oestrogens by no means avoids systemic effects. Indeed the use of oestradiol vaginally is one of the best routes to achieve therapeutic levels (Schiff *et al.*, 1977). It is our opinion that oestriol does not offer oestrogen benefits without the risks, since extremely high oral doses are necessary to circumvent its rapid conjugation by the liver (Schiff *et al.*, 1980b).

RISKS OF OESTROGEN THERAPY

A firm association between the use of oestrogens for the menopause and endometrial cancer has been established: firstly by descriptive studies which demonstrate a clear correlation between recent fluctuations in endometrial cancer incidence and oestrogen sales (Jick *et al.*, 1979) and secondly, by numerous case–control studies of endometrial cancer and menopausal oestrogens (Smith *et al.*, 1975; Ziel and Finkle, 1975; Mack *et al.*, 1976; Gray *et al.*, 1977; McDonald *et al.*, 1977; Antunes *et al.*, 1979; Shapiro *et al.*, 1980). The association has been consistently found and is strong – about a five-fold increase in risk for endometrial cancer from the use of menopausal oestrogens.

Certain biases could have falsely elevated the risk ratios reported but are unlikely to have led to an entirely spurious result. In favour of the association being valid is the fact that a dose-response is seen. Risk increases about 75% with each year of use but drops sharply with discontinuation of use (Cramer and Knapp, 1979). Also the association makes biological sense in that the other major risk factors for endometrial cancer, including ovarian and adrenal tumours, obesity and even liver disease, are all conditions which lead to an excess of oestrogen relative to progesterone (Cramer, 1980).

We should emphasize that the endometrial cancers that arise in the setting of oestrogen therapy are lower in stage and grade and have a very favourable prognosis (Silverberg *et al.*, 1980). Furthermore it would appear that the addition of a progestin to the oestrogen regimen would decrease the risk for endometrial cancer. This is suggested by studies which indicate a protective effect of combination oral contraceptives against endometrial cancer (Weiss and Sayvetz, 1980) and by studies which demonstrate a low incidence of endometrial hyperplasia in women on oestrogen and progesterone combinations (Whitehead, 1978; Thom *et al.*, 1979).

Concerning the risk for breast cancer from menopausal oestrogens, there have been numerous case–control and cohort studies performed (Mustacchi and Gordan, 1958; Wallach and Henneman, 1959; Boston Collaborative Drug Surveillance Program, 1974; Burch *et al.*, 1975; Casagrande *et al.*, 1976; Hoover *et al.*, 1976; Sartwell *et al.*, 1977; Gambrell, 1979; Jick *et al.*, 1980; Ross *et al.*, 1980). The majority done before 1976 have been negative but can be criticized because of failure to correct for confounders such as type of menopause, age at menopause, parity, and age at first birth. Some recent studies of high quality have suggested an increased risk for breast cancer particularly in women with a natural menopause (Jick *et al.*, 1980, Ross *et al.*, 1980).

Taken together, the epidemiologic studies have not shown a strong or consistent association between menopausal oestrogen use and breast cancer. But expect to see continued studies on this subject. It would not be at all surprising to find increased risk for breast cancer in certain subgroups of oestrogen users.

Finally we merely mentioned the possible link between oestrogens and a certain type of ovarian cancer – endometrioid and clear cell cancer (Cramer *et al.*, 1981) – and a possible link between oestrogen therapy and gall-bladder disease (Boston Collaborative Drug Surveillance Program, 1974).

WEIGHING RISKS AND BENEFITS

A randomized clinical trial to clearly demonstrate the benefits or risks of oestrogen therapy is probably not within the realm of feasibility (Hulka *et al.*, 1978). It appears that one must examine the balance between risks and benefits indirectly from so called cost–benefit or cost–effectiveness analysis. Costs of therapy include not only the cost of the drug itself but also the cost of the medical visits and tests that may be necessary for surveillance of ill-effects while on the drug. It also includes costs that may be associated with treating adverse effects that develop. Under benefits are counted the savings associated with the drug's ability to prevent other illnesses, and the value of the net years of life gained (or lost) by the therapy. However it is difficult to place a dollar value on the years of life lost or gained, and difficult to enter quality of life considerations into the equation.

Problems notwithstanding, one economist performed cost–effectiveness analysis with regard to oestrogen therapy and found that it was favourable in women not at risk for endometrial cancer (in women

141

without a uterus) but of only marginal value in women at risk for endometrial cancer (Weinstein, 1980). The analysis may be criticized for failure to take into consideration the effect that different therapeutic regimens (adding progesterone) might have on the risk for endometrial cancer. Thus the decision to use oestrogen therapy is still best left to the judgement of the informed patient and the experienced clinician.

We believe, however, that epidemiologic studies can be used to favourably improve the risk–benefit equation. First, prospective epidemiologic studies can identify the best oestrogen and progesterone regimen to use, and define appropriate medical screening for women on such therapy. Second, epidemiologic studies can be used to identify those women most likely to benefit and those women most likely to suffer risks of oestrogen therapy. For example, the thin, nulliparous woman with an early menopause is likely to suffer osteoporosis and may thus have the most to gain from oestrogen therapy. Concerning risks, some studies would suggest that women with prior benign breast disease may suffer an increased risk for breast cancer from oestrogen (Ross *et al.,* 1980). Finally, since both the complications of the menopause and menopausal therapy increase with time, we propose that epidemiologic studies of the preventable causes of premature menopause be undertaken.

We regard this question of the risks and benefits of replacement therapy as an unfinished story for which we write a new chapter every 3 years. The risks have received attention recently but the balance can be restored by reading what has been written before and carefully applying scientific and epidemiologic principles in our new investigations.

References

Albrecht, B. H., Schiff, I., Tulchinsky, D. and Ryan, K. J. (1981). Objective evidence that placebo and oral medroxyprogesterone acetate therapy diminish menopausal vasomotor flushes. *Am. J. Obstet. Gynecol.,* **139**, 631

Antunes, C. M. F., Stolley, P. D., Rosenshein, N. B., Davies, J. L., Tonascia, J. A., Brown, C., Burnett, L., Rutledge, A., Pokempner, M. and Garcia, R. (1979). Endometrial cancer and estrogen use. Reports of a large case–control study. *N. Engl. J. Med.,* **300**, 9

Boston Collaborative Drug Surveillance Program, Boston University Medical Center (1974). Surgically confirmed gallbladder disease, venous thromboembolism, and breast tumors in relation to post-menopausal estrogen therapy. *N. Engl. J. Med.,* **290**, 15

Bradley, D. D., Wingerd, J., Petitti, D. B., Krauss, R. M. and Ramcharan, S. (1978). Serum high-density-lipoprotein cholesterol in women using oral contraceptives, estrogens and progestins. *N. Engl. J. Med.,* **288**, 17

Burch, J. C., Byrd, B. F. and Vaughn, W. K. (1975). The effects of long-term estrogen administration to women following hysterectomy. In van Keep, P. A. and Lauritzen, C. (eds.). *Estrogens in the Post-Menopause*. Frontiers in Hormone Research. vol. 3, pp. 208–14. (Basel: Karger)

Campbell, S. (1976). Double blind psychometric studies on the effects of natural estrogens on post-menopausal women. In Campbell, S. (ed.). *The Management of the Menopause and Post-menopausal Years*, pp. 149–58. (Baltimore: University Park Press)

Casagrande, J., Gerkins, V., Henderson, B. E., Mach, T. and Pike, M. C. (1976). Brief communications: exogenous estrogens and breast cancer in women with natural menopause. *J. Natl. Cancer Inst.*, **56**, 839

Coope, J. (1976). Double blind cross-over study of estrogen replacement therapy. In Campbell, S. (ed.). *The Management of the Menopause and Post-menopausal Years*, pp. 159–68. (Baltimore: University Park Press)

Coronary Drug Project Research Group (1970). The Coronary Drug Project. Initial findings leading to modifications of its research protocol. *J. Am. Med. Assoc.*; **214**, 1303

Cramer, D. (1980). Epidemiology of endometrial cancer. In Koss, L. G. (ed.). Recent advances in endometrial neoplasia. *Acta Cytol.*, **24**, 478

Cramer, D. W., Devesa, S. S. and Welch, W. R. (1981). Trends in the incidence of endometrioid and clear cell cancer of the ovary in the United States. *Am. J. Epidemiol.*, **114**, 201

Cramer, D. W. and Knapp, R. C. (1979). Review of epidemiologic studies of endometrial cancer and exogenous estrogen. *Obstet. Gynecol.*, **54**, 521

Furman, R. H. (1971). Coronary heart disease and the menopause. In Ryan, K. J. and Gibson, D. C. (eds.). Publication no. 73–319, p. 39. United States Department of Health, Education and Welfare

Gallagher, J. C. and Nordin, B. E. C. (1974). Calcium metabolism and the menopause. In Curry, A. S. and Hewitt, J. V. (eds.). *Biochemistry of Women: Clinical Concepts*, pp 145–75. (Cleveland: CRC)

Gambrell, R. D. (1979). The role of hormones in the etiology of breast and endometrial cancer. *Acta Obstet. Gynecol. Scand. Suppl.*, **88**, 73

Gray, L. A., Christopherson, W. M. and Hoover, R. N. (1977). Estrogens and endometrial carcinoma. *Obstet. Gynecol.*, **49**, 385

Hammond, C. B., Jelovsek, F. R., Lee, K. L., Creasman, W. T. and Parker, R. T. (1979). Effects of long-term estrogen replacement therapy. I. Metabolic effects. *Am. J. Obstet. Gynecol.*, **133**, 525

Hoover, R., Gray, L. A., Cole, P. and MacMahon, B. (1976). Menopausal estrogens and breast cancer. *N. Engl. J. Med.*, **295**, 401

Hulka, B. S., Hogue, C. J. R. and Greenberg, B. G. (1978). Methodologic issues in epidemiologic studies of endometrial cancer and exogenous estrogen. *Am. J. Epidemiol.*, **107**, 267

Hutchinson, T. A., Polansky, S. M. and Feinstein, A. R. (1979). Post-menopausal oestrogens protect against fractures of hip and distal radius. *Lancet*, **2**, 705

Jick, H., Walker, A. M., Watkins, R. N., D'Ewart, D. C., Hunter, J. R., Danford, A., Madsen, S., Dinan, B. J. and Rothman, K. J. (1980). Replacement estrogens and breast cancer. *Am. J. Epidemiol.*, **112**, 586

Jick, H., Watkins, R. N., Hunter, J. R., Dinan, B. J., Madsen, S., Rothman, K. J. and Walker, A. M. (1979). Replacement estrogens and endometrial cancer. *N. Engl. J. Med.*, **300**, 218

Lindsay, R., Aitken, J. M., Anderson, J. B., Hart, D. M., MacDonald, E. B. and Clarke, A. C. (1976). Long-term prevention of post-menopausal osteoporosis by oestrogen. *Lancet*, **1**, 1038

McDonald, T. W., Annegers, J. F., O'Fallon, W. M., Dockerty, M. B., Malkasian,

143

G. D. and Kurland, L. T. (1977). Exogenous estrogen and endometrial carcinoma: case–control and incidence study. *Am. J. Obstet. Gynecol.,* **127**, 572

Mack, T. M., Pike, M. C., Henderson, B. E., Pfeffer, R. I., Gerkins, V. R., Arthur, M. and Brown, S. E. (1976). Estrogens and endometrial cancer in a retirement community. *N. Engl. J. Med.,* **294**, 1262

Mustacchi, P. and Gordan, G. S. (1958). Frequency of cancer in estrogen-treated osteoporotic women. In Segaloff, A. (ed.). *Breast Cancer. The Second Biennial Louisiana Cancer Conference,* pp. 163–9. (St. Louis: Mosby)

Nachtigall, L. E., Nachtigall, R. H., Nachtigall, R. D. and Beckman, E. M. (1979). Estrogen replacement therapy. I. A 10-year prospective study in the relationship to osteoporosis. *Obstet. Gynecol.,* **53**, 277

Nordin, B. E. C. (1971). Clinical significance and pathogenesis of osteoporosis. *Br. Med. J.,* **1**, 571

Pfeffer, R. I., Whipple, G. H., Kurosaki, T. T. and Chapman, J. M. (1978). Coronary risk and estrogen use in post-menopausal woman. *Am. J. Epidemiol.,* **107**, 479

Rosenberg, L., Armstrong, B., Phil, D. and Jick, H. (1976). Myocardial infarction and estrogen therapy in post-menopausal women. *N. Engl. J. Med.,* **294**, 1256

Ross, R. K., Paganini-Hill, A., Gerkins, V. R., Mack, T. M., Pfeffer, R., Arthur, M. and Henderson, B. E. (1980). A case–control study of menopausal estrogen therapy and breast cancer. *J. Am. Med. Assoc.,* **243**, 1635

Ross, R. K., Paganini-Hill, A., Mack, T. M., Arthur, M. and Henderson B. E. (1981). Menopausal oestrogen therapy and protection from death from ischaemic heart disease. *Lancet,* **1**, 858

Ryan, K. J. (1976). Estrogen and atherosclerosis. *Clin. Obstet. Gynecol.,* **19**, 805

Sartwell, P. E., Arthes, F. G. and Tonascia, J. A. (1977). Exogenous hormones, reproductive history and breast cancer. *J. Natl. Cancer Inst.,* **59**, 1589

Schiff, I., Regestein, Q., Tulchinsky, D. and Ryan, K. J. (1979). Effects of estrogens on sleep and psychological state of the hypogonadal woman. *J. Am. Med. Assoc.,* **242**, 2405

Schiff, I., Tulchinsky, D., Cramer, D. and Ryan, K. J. (1980a). Oral medroxyprogesterone treatment of post-menopausal symptoms. *J. Am. Med. Assoc.,* **244**, 1443

Schiff, I., Tulchinsky, D. and Ryan, K. J. (1977). Vaginal absorption of estrone and estradiol-17β. *Fertil. Steril.,* **131**, 585

Schiff, I., Tulchinsky, D., Ryan, K. J., Kadner, S. and Levitz, M. (1980b). Plasma estriol and its conjugates following administration of estriol to post-menopausal women: correlations with gonadotropin levels. *Am. J. Obstet. Gynecol.,* **138**, 1137

Shapiro, S., Kaufman, D. W., Slone, D., Rosenberg, L., Miettinen, O. S., Stolley, P. D., Rosenshein, N. B., Watring, W. G., Leavitt, T. and Knapp, R. C. (1980). Recent and past use of conjugated estrogens in relation to adenocarcinoma of the endometrium. *N. Engl. J. Med.,* **303**, 485

Silverberg, S. G., Mullen, D., Faraci, J. A., Makowski, E. L., Miller, A., Finch, J. L. and Sutherland, J. V. (1980). Endometrial carcinoma: clinical–pathological comparison of cases in post-menopausal women receiving and not receiving exogenous estrogens. *Cancer,* **45**, 3018

Smith, D. C., Prentice, R., Thompson, D. J. and Herrmann, W. L. (1975). Association of exogenous estrogen and endometrial carcinoma. *N. Engl. J. Med.,* **293**, 1164

Thom, M. H., White, P. J., Sturdee, D. W., Paterson, M. E. L. and Studd, J. W. W. (1979). Prevention and treatment of endometrial disease in climacteric women receiving oestrogen therapy. *Lancet,* **2**, 455

Wallach, S. and Henneman, P. H. (1959). Prolonged estrogen therapy in post-menopausal women. *J. Am. Med. Assoc.,* **171**, 1637

Weinstein, M. C. (1980). Estrogen use in post-menopausal women – Costs, risks and benefits. *N. Engl. J. Med.*, **303**, 308

Weiss, N. S. and Sayvetz, T. A. (1980). Incidence of endometrial cancer in relation to use of oral contraceptives. *N. Engl. J. Med.*, **302**, 551

Weiss, N. S., Ure, C. L., Ballard, J. H., Williams, A. R. and Daling, J. R. (1980). Decreased risk of fractures of the hip and lower forearm with post-menopausal use of estrogen. *N. Engl. J. Med.*, **303**, 1195

Whitehead, M. I. (1978). The effects of oestrogens and progestogens on the post-menopausal endometrium. *Maturitas*, **1**, 87

Ziel, H. K. and Finkle, W. D. (1975). Increased risk of endometrial carcinoma among users of conjugated estrogens. *N. Engl. J. Med.*, **293**, 1167

Workshop 15

Menopause clinics: purpose, function and international comparisons

---

Moderator: **W. H. Utian** (USA)

Speakers: **T. Abe** (Japan)
             C. van der Does (The Netherlands)
             M. Flint (USA)
             C. Gold (Canada)
             J. Hailes (Australia)
             B. Maoz (Israel)
             J. Need (Australia)
             M. Notelovitz (USA)
             I. van Seumeren (The Netherlands)
             M. Smith (Australia)
             D. Sturdee (UK)
             A. Vizzotto (Italy)
             M. I. Whitehead (UK)
             B. Wren (Australia)

INTRODUCTION

During the Second International Congress on the Menopause, which was held in Jerusalem in 1978, an informal session was conducted on menopause clinics. This meeting was so successful that the organizing committee decided that a full session should be devoted to this subject at the Ostend Congress. On this occasion it was generally conceded that much headway had been made in defining the implications of menopause and its treatment, but that more needed to be done in terms of delivering this information and therapy directly to women.

The value of a menopause clinic for the centralization and control of oestrogen therapy was first described by Utian (1977 and 1979). His Groote Schuur Hospital Menopause Clinic, the first menopause research clinic in the world, was highly successful in stimulating inter-disciplinary long-term collaborative research, and served as a rôle model for later descriptions of the values of such clinics. In summary the benefits of a menopause clinic are as follows:

(1) It serves as a well woman's clinic for middle-aged and older females. As a natural progression from family planning and prenatal programmes, an opportunity is created to provide medical check-ups for women of older age groups who may not otherwise be offered such services.

(2) Screening programmes for breast cancer, diabetes, hypertension, etc., can be introduced and co-ordinated for large populations.

(3) Menopause experience is gathered in one centre.

(4) All medical and paramedical specialties (e.g., psychiatry, internal medicine, sociology, dietetics, etc.) can be involved and coordinated.

(5) Oestrogen therapy can be better controlled and evaluated on a short- or long-term basis. In particular, the long-term benefits and risks of such therapy can be more effectively observed.

(6) Centralization of care can be made extremely cost-effective.

(7) A menopause service can offer broad educational programmes with a potential for better informing the patient, and contributing to changed societal attitudes as well.

(8) Small or large group counselling, including self-help programmes, can be initiated and directed on a wide geographic basis.

(9) Research is a major component of a menopause clinic, and a specialized clinic is best able to carry out long-term evaluations of the effects of various hormone treatments.

The team of international authorities invited to participate in the present workshop on menopause clinics was asked to consider the following aspects:

(1) Need and availability of clinics.

(2) Scope and purpose.

(3) Base – hospital or outside?

(4) Staffing – medical, paramedical, and other.

(5) Data gathering – clinic forms, computerization, etc.

(6) Methods of informing public of existence and purpose.

(7) Educational and out-reach programmes.

(8) Research rôle.

(9) Clinic operation.

ABSTRACTS OF REPORTS BY NATIONALITY

Australia

Need reported that Australia has a menopause clinic attached to teaching hospitals in each capital city and a few others based in community health centres. Clinics are necessary in order to provide advice and hormone replacement therapy (HRT) withheld by many general practitioners, and to supervise such treatment. Such clinics distinguish psychosocial from oestrogen withdrawal symptoms and undertake research. Hospital-based clinics treat a highly selected population with a high incidence of psychosomatic symptoms. *Need* feels that menopause clinics should ideally be staffed by medical personnel with counselling skills in social aspects, and by a social worker or community health nurse who can undertake group work. Research functions should define and tabulate symptoms directly related to oestrogen withdrawal, assess the real risk of oestrogen treatment as far as endometrial cancer is concerned, explore the efficacy of progestogens and their regimen in preventing endometrial cancer, note effects on cholesterol metabolism, and examine the rôle of HRT in preventing the later development of osteoporosis. She feels that there are disadvantages as well as advantages in the clinics being hospital-based.

Hailes reported that two menopause clinics in Victoria, Australia, are based within hospitals and are directly accessible to the public without

149

referral, due to the resistance of many practitioners towards hormonal therapy. Both clinics are heavily booked, and patient care is integrated with research projects. Mature female staff are found to be most successful. Other departments within the hospital are freely available for referral. The public is informed of the clinics' work by press articles, radio programmes, literature and medical lectures to women's groups. Undergraduate and postgraduate teaching is conducted in the units.

Smith explained that Perth, West Australia, has a population of 1.25 million, of whom some 166 000 are women over 45. Perth is geographically isolated from the rest of Australia, and the problems encountered there tend to differ somewhat from those found in Melbourne and Sydney. Until 1979 menopause problems were handled by general practitioners or by gynaecologists, many of whom were reluctant to prescribe oestrogen therapy. They were also reluctant to refer patients to a special clinic when, through public pressure, one was established. Only when Professor B. E. C. Nordin from Leeds in the United Kingdom provided discrete 'advertising' as a visiting professor did the clinic begin to flourish. It has now developed into a hormone replacement therapy clinic with research interests; it is, for example, attempting to determine the smallest dose of oestrogen required to relieve symptoms and to protect against osteoporosis, and is also investigating the use of progestogens alone in high-risk cases.

Wren spoke of the three-fold purpose of clinics: patient care, teaching, and research. He listed the planning steps which must be considered before opening a menopause clinic, and gave a brief outline of the reasons for and consequences of setting up such a clinic. The needs, aims, objectives, and planning steps were discussed and, as a model, he gave a summary of the events which led to the establishment of the menopause clinic at the Royal Hospital for Women in Paddington, New South Wales. He also described two questionnaires and a patient information sheet which, he felt, could be used as a basis for developing similar material for use in other menopause clinics; a point which was developed further during the general discussion.

Canada

Gold explained that in Toronto the Mature Woman's Clinic functions within the Department of Obstetrics and Gynecology of Toronto General Hospital, and is affiliated with the Department of Obstetrics and Gynecology at the University of Toronto. When opened in April 1980 it was the first unit in Canada which cared specifically for the needs of women in the climacteric. The clinic provides patient care on a doctor-referred or self-referred basis. It is active in undergraduate and post-graduate teaching, research, and speaking to professional and non-professional groups.

Canada has a universally-available, government health-care insurance programme. It is important to note that university departments and hospital departments all have to operate within annual individual budgets. If a new service, such as a Mature Woman's Clinic is to be added, the funds have to be found within the Department of Obstetrics and Gynecology, and may mean that some other services have to be withdrawn. Funding is a very difficult problem.

Obstetrics and Gynecology is a surgical sub-specialty in Canada. A gynaecologist spending 45 minutes with a patient will receive a lower fee for his services than would an internal medicine specialist. The operation of a diagnostic medical-gynaecology (non-surgical) clinic, such as a menopause clinic, cannot be self-supporting within the health insurance programme. Outside support is needed.

Israel

Maoz reported that at present there are no menopause clinics in Israel, but that several studies have been conducted in an attempt to find out just what sort of service should be offered in this respect. These studies have led to the conclusion that the desired model is a multi-disciplinary one. The first study indicated (a) that climacteric symptoms should be assessed in terms of general health evaluation, and (b) that the symptoms are caused and shaped partly by psycho-social and cultural factors. The second study showed the importance of good collaboration between gynaecological and psychiatric teams – a once problematical and disappointing relationship – and the third emphasized the need to include the husbands in the evaluation process and treatment of the climacteric of their wives.

Italy

Vizzotto reported that the organization of menopause clinics is one of the main interests of the recently formed Italian Menopause Society. A few clinics are already operational: one in Bologna, two in Milan, one in Turin, and one in Rome.

Some common problems have been recognized. It is already clear that admission criteria need to be well-defined. Patients who ask for help at a menopause clinic should be 'screened' before being accepted for treatment, with factors such as chronological age, menstrual pattern, and climacteric symptoms being taken into account.

It is felt that a common data sheet for use in all menopause clinics would be helpful, partly because it would aid the development of a common policy. Such forms would also facilitate the conducting of multi-centre studies, which would be particularly welcome in Italy as they would permit a comparison of different geographic and social environments.

Menopause clinics need a multi-disciplinary approach, but specialists should be chosen according to the local problems and facilities. The gynaecologist remains the key person, other specialists – cardiologists and radiologists, for example – being required on a consultant basis.

The Italian menopause clinics have two main aims: (a) to provide a comprehensive approach to the patients' health care, and (b) to facilitate the conducting of clinical trials and of scientific research.

Japan

Abe described his clinic in Japan. This is a menopause clinic established within the Department of Obstetrics and Gynaecology of Tohoku University Hospital in Sendai. Since its opening in 1971, the clinic has dealt with the climacteric syndromes of approximately 800 patients. Most of the patients have been between 35 and 55 years in age, about one-third being post-artificial menopause. This clinic performs evaluations of the endocrine profile and of the complaints of patients, in an attempt to clarify the mechanism of the onset of the climacteric syndrome. This leads to a differentiation between endocrine and psychiatric symptoms, and therefore to the prescribing of more precise and appropriate treatments.

The Netherlands

Experience in Leiden demonstrates the problems likely to be faced in the establishment of a *regional menopause programme*, as opposed to a specific menopause clinic. *Van der Does* stressed that before embarking upon a regional extramural health care project, agreement should be reached between all participants on the ultimate goals of the project. Gynae-cologists of the three hospitals in Leiden noted considerable confusion concerning the complaints of the climacteric and the use of oestrogens by the general practitioners of the town and region. At a meeting convened to discuss these matters, it was decided that an intramural department out-patient menopause clinic was probably not advisable. The preferred alternative was a regional programme to treat patients with specific complaints at the peripheral level. The complaints and treatment modalities were specifically determined by a protocol devised especially for these circumstances.

The goals of the co-operative project of the regional general practitioners and the gynaecologists of the three hospitals were:

(1) To supply information concerning the climacteric to the general practitioner.

(2) To bring some unity in the various individual methods of treatment.

(3) To ascertain certain groups at risk.

(4) To study the most predominant symptoms mentioned by the patients.

(5) To ascertain the awareness of the doctor to pick up climacteric symptoms which may be masked by vague complaints.

At the outset, the service side of the project tended to be confused with the research side of it, each component presenting its own problems. The requirements for clinical service are totally different to the collection of reliable data for research. This led to physician frustration and a high rate of physician drop-out. Regular meetings, at least one every half year, helped remedy the situation; twenty general practitioners of the original sixty are still participating in the project. The question of whether some doctors feel that their knowledge of the subject has been sufficiently enhanced to allow them to continue on their own is under investigation.

Van Seumeren at the University of Utrecht described the experience of the first hospital menopause clinic in the Netherlands. The team there is multi-disciplinary. The secretary and nurse are considered very important, often giving advice by telephone. The purpose of the clinic is similar to that of the other hospital-based clinics mentioned in this report, and the clinic in Utrecht has a large research component.

United Kingdom

Sturdee reported that the computer recording of data from women attending a menopause clinic has allowed a much more detailed analysis than would otherwise be possible. In particular, this has provided further elucidation of the symptomatology of the climacteric and correlation between individual symptoms and groups of symptoms. The addition of results from routine biochemical screening has demonstrated some correlations of symptoms with biochemical parameters of liver function, and the monitoring of serum biochemical change in post-menopausal women receiving oestrogen–progestogen therapy has also been possible by discriminant function analysis. He emphasized that all patients are seen only by referral from the general practitioner.

Whitehead discussed menopause clinics in broad perspective in the United Kingdom. There are 21 such clinics in the UK at the present time. In 1980 these clinics dealt with approximately 2500 new patients (calculated from Medical Research Council returns). It is estimated that the clinics continued to supervise some 12 000 patients who were first registered in previous years, and thus, nationally, menopause clinics may be said to be performing approximately 3–4% of the total potential workload, estimated at about 400 000 women. More clinics are obviously needed.

The geographic location of menopause clinics is also less than ideal. Although there are seven clinics in London, in the area west of Oxford to Cornwall there are none at all. Patients in poorly served regions have to travel long distances for proper therapy. Only 20% of the patients seen in the King's College Hospital clinic in London live in the immediate vicinity of the hospital.

Because of excessive demands and insufficient funding, the majority of menopause clinics in the UK have a limited scope and provide only a clinical service. Eight of the clinics, however, are currently engaged in active research programmes, and the data that are generated appear to be fairly rapidly disseminated back to the general practitioners. The most effective routes of communication are evening lectures, film shows, and articles in the medical press. The teaching out-reach would be considerably improved if the pharmaceutical industry representatives (who see general practitioners regularly) were also kept abreast of the most recent developments; *Whitehead* feels that the lack of knowledge displayed by some is quite appalling.

The research, most of which is undertaken by the larger units, usually takes the form of prospective studies involving small numbers of patients. Large scale epidemiological investigations, comparable with those reported in American literature, are underway but patient recruitment has been disappointing because the use of oestrogens in the general population in the UK is very low. Some epidemiologists have openly expressed doubts about the cost:effectiveness of epidemiological studies on this subject in the UK. Most current research programmes rely heavily on technology and good laboratory back-up. Whilst these programmes are valuable, there is scope for research in areas requiring less technical support; for example, in an assessment of progestin effects on the symptomatic and psychological status. Better co-ordinated research programmes between clinics would undoubtedly be fruitful, but these are unlikely until staff from different clinics begin communicating with one another. At present, cross-pollination is zero.

United States of America

Flint described a different model for menopause care. This is a private menopause programme, named Mid-Life Challenge, which accepts referrals from physicians, therapists and others. Unlike a menopause clinic *per se*, which has physicians associated with it, this programme refers back to the physicians, if necessary, patients participating in either the three-week or six-week regimen which it offers. Basically an educational programme, Mid-Life Challenge offers peer counselling, a customized exercise regimen, nutritional consultation with a diet tailored to each client's needs, and instruction in relaxation techniques. Menopause is only one of the topics discussed in each peer counselling session. Problems of middle-age, such as returning to the job market, the care of ageing parents, becoming single again, setting new life goals, improving one's well-being, etc., are covered in group discussions. Group support, referrals, and education about the 'ageing' process, including menopause, combined with nutrition advice and exercise, make this a holistic approach to the care of women in mid-life, whether pre-menopausal, peri-menopausal or post-menopausal.

Notelovitz also spoke of the importance of an holistic approach being adopted by a climacteric centre, the objectives of which should be service, education, and research. He recommended that such a centre should include a 'menopause' clinic, a hormone replacement facility, a 'well-ness' laboratory, a physical fitness and nutrition counselling service, a urodynamic clinic, and counselling services on psychological and sexual aspects, occupational therapy, and mid-life professional opportunities. He emphasized the need for specially-trained professionals to supply these services and discussed the development of 'climacteric physicians', a type of specialist general practitioner, and of appropriately trained nurses and paramedical staff.

GENERAL DISCUSSION

(1) Need and availability of clinics

There still exists a remarkable paucity of epidemiological data on community needs for menopause clinics, for ancillary services such as group counselling, and for large-scale regional programmes. Fortunately, the awareness engendered in recent years has lead to the introduction of preliminary demographic data gathering, and there is hope that substantial advances will soon be forthcoming.

The general consensus of opinion in this workshop was that menopause clinics should be an integral part of community health programmes. There is a specific need for them, particularly in middle and lower income communities where private medical care is not easily available. Not surprisingly therefore, the development of menopause clinics to date has been stronger in countries with some degree of socialized medicine.

(2) Scope and purpose

The scope and purpose of menopause clinics has been outlined in the general introduction to this workshop report. The following were also considered to be areas of importance:

  (a) a service to patients
  (b) a means of disseminating information regarding the menopause
  (c) a source of patients for research into menopause
  (d) a means of teaching medical and paramedical staff.

(3) Base – hospital or outside?

Traditionally, if one may use such a term in this connection, menopause clinics have been established within university teaching hospitals, and documented descriptions of such clinics have to date related only to this type of service (*Utian*, 1977, 1979 and 1980a). The current meeting was of particular interest in that other types of services were described, and considerable controversy generated. *Flint* outlined an ancillary type of menopause service, one not under the direct control of a medical practitioner, but acting instead as a paramedical service; *Van der Does* discussed a comprehensive approach to the development of a regional service through the general practitioners; *Notelovitz* described virtually an expanded new specialty with a super-general practitioner titled a 'climacteric physician' interrelating with a full range of specialists. These various alternatives highlight the fact that different solutions are necessary for different communities. The common factor is that the services described have been of value.

The ideal solution would seem to be the following:

(1) Primary care being conducted through general practitioners, preferably under the direction and co-ordination of the tertiary care (high-risk) centre.

(2) Supportive care offered through paramedical services, possibly of the model described by *Flint*, i.e., a service analogous to the natural childbirth classes conducted in obstetrics.

(3) Tertiary control conducted through teaching hospital menopause clinics. The latter would thus be responsible for the care of referral cases rather than primary care, and would also direct the research and educational components of menopause care.

(4) Staffing – medical, paramedical and other

Decisions on staffing the clinic will depend on the major purpose of the clinic, as previously specified. *Wren* emphasized that if the clinic is to be purely a service clinic, then only gynaecologists will be required, and information need only be recorded on routine clinic notes. If, however, the clinic is to serve another specific purpose then the staff needed to achieve this purpose must be employed. Psychologists with their special skills and counselling techniques may play a major rôle; endocrinologists, psychiatrists, etc., may be regarded as integral to the clinic and provision must be made to have these members available at every session. It is also important that the clinic have access to other interested medical and paramedical specialists. Thus, dependent upon individual patient needs, easy referral patterns need to be established.

Experience at the Groote Schuur Hospital Menopause Clinic has highlighted the need for a top quality secretary and/or social worker to be engaged. Such an individual is extremely helpful for the co-ordination of services, and as a direct contact person with whom the patient may communicate at all times during the working week.

(5) Data gathering – clinic forms, computerization, etc.

For routine clinics, brief medical notes by a gynaecologist may be all that is necessary. If research is to be undertaken, however, a far more detailed and precise recording system is called for. This may proceed through a computerized system. A decision must therefore be made before the clinic begins, and if research is to be a major component of the clinic, a comprehensive questionnaire and system of recording all facts must be developed. The availability of computer facilities is ideal.

An unresolved question related to whether questionnaires should be of the self-assessment or physician-completed type. A co-ordination of both would probably be ideal.

Wren of Australia described the questionnaire used at the Royal Hospital for Women in Paddington. Further discussion led to a general consensus that, although perhaps difficult to achieve, an 'International Menopause Clinic Questionnaire' would be ideal. *Utian* offered to attempt to correlate the forms presently used around the world and to produce a computer-compatible 'International Form' for discussion at the next congress. Participants at the workshop were requested to forward their clinic forms to him for this purpose. The value of an 'International Form' as a tool for cross-cultural studies would be considerable.

(6) Methods of informing the public of clinic services

Several methods were outlined for publicizing the existence of a menopause clinic. Variations in local situations will of course limit the value of some of the following:

(a) an internal hospital memorandum
(b) announcement letter to general practitioners, gynaecologists, psychiatrists, and community health services
(c) general media publicity – the press and television
(d) advertising.

(7) Educational and out-reach programmes

Such a vast volume of *misinformation* is available to the public that it is not surprising that many women are confused about the menopause, and that numerous misconceptions persist.

Education was thus considered by the panel to be a major objective of a menopause clinic. In this respect, education was sub-divided into that directed at the general public and that more specifically devised for the medical profession. The educational component should comprise both an internal programme for clinic participants and an out-reach programme for the community. This out-reach programme should comprise a panel of speakers with topics that can be delivered both to professional and to lay audiences.

It was considered advisable for each clinic to produce a brochure pertinent to local circumstances. Additional information could be provided through the distribution of carefully screened booklets produced by the pharmaceutical industry. For those patients wanting more detailed information, reference could be made to books written for the lay public but based on currently acceptable research data (*Utian* 1978 and 1980b).

(8) Research rôle

A tertiary care teaching hospital-based clinic was considered to be the ideal centre for research, but not the only one. Certainly, metabolic studies would generally be limited to the hospital-based clinics, but demographic research and drug trials could be directed through regional programmes. The general consensus of the panel was that every clinic should attempt *some* research, and that the key to this was a good record and follow-up system.

(9) Clinic operation

Skilful planning is necessary if a clinic is to operate successfully. Areas discussed included the following:

(a) importance of a strict and adequate appointment system
(b) screening of patients – who should attend the clinic?
(c) first contact with clinic staff
(d) telephone communication and follow-up questions
(e) self-completed versus staff-completed questionnaires for history-taking
(f) physical examinations – minimal and optimal procedures
(g) special tests – diagnostic and/or research (an exact plan is extremely important)
(h) control of therapy – the use of specific protocols is of importance; the question of fixed dosages versus flexible individualization of therapy was debated
(i) follow-up visits – frequency and procedures
(j) follow-up of abnormal test results
(k) referrals to other services
(l) distribution of educational material

(m) fiscal details – funding, direct costs to patients, pharmaceutical costs, etc.

CONCLUSIONS

The understanding and treatment of the female climacteric has entered a new phase. Specifically, there now appears sufficient justification to warrant the establishment of regionalized programmes for climacteric care. Such programmes would appear a logical link between the prenatal and family planning services offered to women of reproductive age, and the general services offered later to the geriatric patient.

These climacteric services would involve general health screening programmes, therapy for the climacteric syndrome, research into current therapeutic modalities and newer concepts, and demographic studies to better identify both the population at risk and the actual incidence of specific risk factors.

There is no ideal model at present, nor is one model likely to satisfy all needs, the health structure varying greatly in different parts of the world. Nonetheless, many of the ideas discussed at this workshop could be applied elsewhere.

There was a general consensus that an 'International Menopause Clinic Questionnaire' was urgently needed to allow for better correlation between clinics, and for cross-cultural comparisons. Participants in this workshop agreed to submit existing forms for incorporation into an 'international form' which, hopefully, will be presented by this workshop chairman at the next International Congress on the Menopause, provisionally planned for 1984.*

Two points stood clear from the discussions which took place during this workshop. The first is that since the menopause clinics began to be established the general understanding both of the lay and of the professional communities regarding the climacteric has been considerably enhanced; the second is that the services provided by the clinics have met with great demand. It is clear that the Menopause Clinic, as an integral part of female health care, has indeed come of age.

---

*Readers who would like to contribute to this project by submitting questionnaires and forms of their own are warmly invited to do so. The material should be sent to Dr W. H. Utian, The Mount Sinai Medical Center of Cleveland, Department of Obstetrics–Gynecology, University Circle, Cleveland, OH 44106, USA.

References

Utian, W. H. (1977). Current status of menopause and postmenopausal estrogen therapy. *Obstet. Gynecol. Survey*, **32**, 193

Utian W. H. (1978). *The Menopause Manual – A Woman's Guide to the Menopause*. (Lancaster: MTP Press)

Utian, W. H. (1979). Estrogen replacement in the menopause. In Wynn, R. M. (ed.). *Obstetrics and Gynecology Annual*, vol. 8. (New York: Appleton)

Utian, W. H. (1980a). *Menopause in Modern Perspective*. (New York: Appleton)

Utian, W. H. (1980b). *Your Middle Years – A Doctor's Guide for Today's Woman*. (New York: Appleton)

Other communications

FREE COMMUNICATIONS

I. Menopause: medical, psychological, epidemiological and social aspects (Chairman: B. Maoz)

Are climacteric symptoms of psychic or hormonal origin?
W. Dmoch (Universitäts–Frauenklinik Düsseldorf, Psychosomatische Abteilung, Moorenstrasse 5, 4000 Düsseldorf, West Germany)

Psycho-endocrine differences and correlations in symptomatic and asymptomatic climacteric women: possible rôle of prolactin.
E. W. W. Sonnendecker, L. Gerdes and E. S. Polakow (E. W. W.S. University of the Witwatersrand, Medical School, Department of Obstetrics and Gynaecology, Johannesburg Hospital, Jubilee Road, Parktown 2193, South Africa)

Psycho-social and health factors of women under 40 following surgical menopause.
M. C. Dougherty, J. L. Resnick, M. Notelovitz and J. Tjapkes (J. L. R., The Center for Climacteric Studies, University of Florida, The Professional Center, 901 NW 8th Avenue, Suite B-1, Gainesville, FL 32601, USA)

Anticipate the menopause.
J. Abrams (Rutgers Medical School, Piscataway, NJ 08854, USA)

Climacteric complaints according to body weight in women of different socio-economic and cultural groups.

C. Campagnoli, G. Morra, P. Belforte, L. Belforte and L. Prelato (C.C., Sezione di Ginecologia Endocrinologica, Ospedale 'Sant' Anna', Corso Spezia 60, 10126 Torino, Italy)

A comparative study of peri-menopausal women self-selecting oestrogen replacement or no drug treatment.

J. L. Resnick, L. Cohen, M. C. Dougherty and M. Notelovitz (J.L.R., The Center for Climacteric Studies, University of Florida, The Professional Center, 901 NW 8th Avenue, Suite B-1, Gainesville, FL 32601, USA)

Menopausal age among various ethnic groups in Israel.

A. Neri, D. Bider, Y. Lidor and Y. Ovadia (A.N., The Beilinson Medical Center, Department of Obstetrics and Gynecology, Petah-Tiqva, Israel)

The effect of hormone replacement therapy on bioelectric potential difference in endometrium, cervix and vagina.

S. L. B. Duncan, P. N. Price and J. Curson (S.L.B.D., University of Sheffield, Department of Obstetrics and Gynaecology, Clinical Sciences Centre, Northern General Hospital, Herries Road, Sheffield S5 7AU, UK)

Psychological consequences of blind drug trials in the treatment of women following surgical menopause.

J. L. Resnick, L. Cohen, M. C. Dougherty, and M. Notelovitz (J.L.R., The Center for Climacteric Studies, University of Florida, The Professional Center, 901 NW 8th Avenue, Suite B-1, Gainesville, FL 32601, USA)

Plasma opioids in spontaneous and surgical menopause.

A. R. Genazzani, F. Facchinetti, D. Parrini, F. Petraglia, M. G. Ricci-Danero and V. Facchini (A.R.G., Università degli Studi di Siena, Cattedra di Patologia Ostetrica e Ginecologica, Via Pietro Mascagni 4, 53100 Siena, Italy)

Effects of two progestogens (norethisterone and dydrogesterone) on lipoproteins in the post-menopause.

A. Netter and E. Laham, (E.L., Université de Beyrouth, Faculté de Médecine, Beyrouth, Lebanon)

Feminine perspectives on the menopause.

J. Willadsen (Copenhagen County Psychiatric Hospital Nordvang, 2600 Glostrup, Denmark)

Breast dysplasias, FSH, LH and PRLH patterns in women taking an oral contraceptive.

J. A. Clavero-Núñez, A. Pereira and A. Villarreal (J.A.C.-N., Servicio I de Obstetricia y Ginecologia, Maternidad Provincial, P. Castellana 122, Madrid 16, Spain)

II. Endocrine aspects (Chairman: R. D. Bulbrook)

Changes in the circadian rhythms of testosterone, LH and PRL with age.

C. Carani, V. Montanini, A. Volpe, A. Baldini, L. Della Casa and P. Marrama (A.V., Università di Modena, Istituto di Clinica Ostetrica e Ginecologica, 41100 Modena, Italy)

Dynamic pattern of gonadotrophins and prolactin in aged men.

V. Montanini, C. Carani, A. Volpe, F. Baraghini, L. Della Casa and P. Marrama (A.V., Università di Modena, Istituto di Clinica Ostetrica e Ginecologica, 41100 Modena, Italy)

Changes in endocrine patterns with age; differences between men and women.

S. Kono, Y. Gibo, T. Nishimura and I. Mori (S.K., Kagoshima University, Faculty of Medicine, Department of Obstetrics and Gynaecology, 1208-1 Usuki-cho, Kagoshima, Japan)

Prolactin, gonadotrophin, and oestrogen levels, and endometrial morphology in women receiving different forms of hormone replacement therapy.

A. Grasso, F. Baraghini, C. Barbieri, E. Dalla Vecchia, G. C. Di Renzo and A. Volpe (A.V., Università di Modena, Istituto di Clinica Ostetrica e Ginecologica, 41100 Modena, Italy)

Plasma androstenedione in pre- and post-menopausal women and in endometrial and ovarian pathology.

P. Scirpa, D. Mango, F. Battaglia, S. Scirpa and A. Montemurro (P.S., Università Cattolica del Sacro Cuore, Facoltà di Medicina, Via della Pineta Sacchetti 644, 00168 Roma, Italy)

Androgens in post-menopausal women: plasma levels of 3alpha-androstanediol.

V. Toscano, F. Abbadessa, E. Fabietti, C. Felicetti, M.-P. Genderini, S. Marini, A. Rovigatti, G. Matarazzo and G. Sorcini (G.S., Università di Roma, Istituto di Clinica Medica Generale e Terapia Medica V, Via Bellinzona 27, Rome, Italy)

A simplified method of measuring androstenedione production rate.
R. G. Crilly, D. H. Marshall and B. E. C. Nordin (B.E.C.N., MRC Mineral Metabolism Unit, The General Infirmary, Great George Street, Leeds LS1 3EX, UK)

Serum hormone parameters in obese women in the post-menopause.
K. Klinga, T. von Holst and B. Runnebaum (K.K., Ruprecht-Karls-Universität Heidelberg, Frauenklinik, Abteilung 8.1.2., Gynäkologische Endokrinologie, Vossstrasse 9, 6900 Heidelberg 1, West Germany)

Body size, sex steroids and their free fractions in patients with endometrial cancer or osteoporotic hip fractures.
B. J. Davidson, L. R. Laufer, J. C. Gambone, R. K. Ross, G. I. Hammond, P. K. Siiteri and H. L. Judd (B.J.D., Loma Linda University, School of Medicine, Department of Gynecology and Obstetrics, Loma Linda Campus, Loma Linda, CA 92350, USA)

The hormonal profile of endometrial carcinoma.
M. Oettinger, A. Mitrani, Y. Zamberg, A. Zilberman and M. Sharf (M.O., Rothschild University Hospital Technion, Faculty of Medicine, Haifa, Israel)

Hormonal parameters of normal pre-menopausal and post-menopausal women, compared to those of patients with uterine bleeding with and without endometrial carcinoma.
T. von Holst, K. Klinga and B. Runnebaum (T.v.H., Ruprecht-Karls-Universität Heidelberg, Frauenklinik, Abteilung 8.1.2., Gynäkologische Endokrinologie, Vossstrasse 9, 6900 Heidelberg 1, West Germany)

Changes of sex-dependent-serum-proteins by menopause.
S. Hashimoto, S. Ishida, T. Harada, E. Nishida and S. Migita (S.H., Kanazawa University School of Medicine, Department of Obstetrics and Gynaecology, Takaramachi 13-1, Kanazawa 920, Japan)

Lipid metabolism with ageing of women.
N. Shinkawa, Y. Unoki, S. Kono and I. Mori (N.S., Kagoshima University,

Faculty of Medicine, Department of Obstetrics and Gynaecology, 1208-1, Usuki-cho, Kagoshima, Japan)

A study of the absorption and metabolism of oral oestrone, oestradiol and oestriol.
G. I. Dyer, P. T. Townsend, O. Young, W. P. Collins and M. I. Whitehead (G.I.D., King's College Hospital Medical School, Department of Obstetrics and Gynaecology, Denmark Hill, London SE5 8RX, UK)

III. Aspects of therapy – general (Chairman: C. Lauritzen)

Intrauterine progesterone contraceptive system (52 mg) in perimenopausal patients with endometrial hyperplasia.
A. Volpe, M. Abrate, E. Dalla Vecchia, M. Mantovani, C. Carani, A. Grasso and V. Mazza (A.V., Università di Modena, Istituto di Clinica Ostetrica e Ginecologica, 41100 Modena, Italy)

On the oestrogen induction of two plasma proteins and the effect of norethisterone.
U.-B. Ottosson, S. Helgason, M.-G. Damber and B. von Schoultz (B.v.S., University of Umeå, Department of Obstetrics and Gynaecology, 901 87 Umeå, Sweden)

Morphological studies of the endometrium during artificial cycles in the post-menopausal woman.
H. Rozenbaum (15 rue Daru, 75008 Paris, France)

Dose-dependency studies on the effects of oestrogen creams.
P. T. Townsend, G. I. Dyer, O. Young, S. Campbell and M. I. Whitehead (P.T.T., King's College Hospital Medical School, Department of Obstetrics and Gynaecology, Denmark Hill, London SE5 8RX, UK)

Clinical, cytological and biological study of intravaginal oestriol (Ortho Gynest) in post-menopausal patients.
S. Wesel (Hôpital de Braine-l'Alleud-Waterloo, 35 rue Wayez, 1420 Braine-l'Alleud, Belgium)

A retrospective study concerning the side effects of long-term oestrogen treatment in climacteric women.
C. Lauritzen and F. Meier (C.L., Universität Ulm, Frauenklinik, Prittwitzstrasse 43, 7900 Ulm/Donau, West Germany)

Long-term effects of progestogen on bone mass in peri-menopausal women.
J. Dequeker and E. De Muylder (J.D., Katholieke Universiteit Leuven, Academisch Ziekenhuis, Weligerveld 1, 3041 Pellenberg, Belgium)

Inter-relationships between oestrogen and the major calcium regulating hormones.
G. Lane, P. T. Townsend, J. Stevenson, C. Hillyard and M. I. Whitehead (G.L., King's College Hospital Medical School, Department of Obstetrics and Gynaecology, Denmark Hill, London SE5 8RX, UK)

Bone mineral content and adrenal steroids in post-menopausal women.
A. Lagrelius, S. Brody, K. Carlström, N.-O. Lunell and L. Rosenborg (A.L., Karolinska Institutet, Department of Obstetrics and Gynaecology, Huddinge Sjukhus, 141 86 Huddinge, Sweden)

Bone mass after withdrawal of oestrogen/gestagen in early post-menopausal females.
C. Christiansen, M. S. Christensen and I. Transbøl (C.C., Glostrup Hospital, Department of Clinical Chemistry, 2600 Glostrup, Denmark)

Bone mineral loss in the axial and appendicular skeleton of oophorecto-mized women.
B. Ettinger, H. K. Genant, C. E. Cann and G. S. Gordan (B.E., The Permanente Medical Group, 2200 O'Farrell Street, San Francisco, CA 94115, USA)

Endocrine and metabolic changes following bilateral oophorectomy and the effect of oestrogen replacement and calcium supplementation.
D. A. Davey, B. L. Cohen, S. Epstein, P. Jacobs, M. Katz, L. Kernoff, B. Pimstone, W. Utian and G. Watermeyer (D.A.D., University of Cape Town Medical School, Department of Obstetrics and Gynaecology, Observatory, 7925 Cape, South Africa)

The carpal tunnel syndrome – A disease typical for the menopause.
M. Arndt and E. Brug (M.A., Chirurgische Universitätsklinik Münster, Jungeblodtplatz 1, 44 Münster, West Germany)

Choice of oestrogen and mode of administration in the therapy of the climacteric.

L. Rauramo (University of Turku, Department of Obstetrics and Gynaecology, Kaskenkatu II B, 20700 Turku 70, Finland)

IV. Aspects of therapy – oestriol (Chairman: D. M. Serr)

The pharmacology of oestriol.
J. van der Vies (Organon International B.V., Endocrinological R & D Laboratories, P.O. Box 20, 5340 BH Oss, The Netherlands)

Effects of oestriol. A clinical view.
P. F. Tauber (Universitätsklinikum Essen, Frauenklinik und Poliklinik, Hufelandstrasse 55, 4300 Essen 1, West Germany)

Comparison of the effects of different dosage regimens of oestriol succinate in the therapy of post-menopausal women.
N. Dombrowicz and P. Delacroix (N.D., Pepermanstraat 9, 4100 Seraing, Belgium)

Assessment of the effect of oestriol-succinate on complex bladder symptoms at the menopause.
C. Richards (Caerphilly District Miners' Hospital, St. Martins Road, Caerphilly CF8 2WW, UK)

Urinary incontinence in 70–75-year-old women; its prevalence, and the effects of oestriol treatment.
G. Samsioe, I. Jansson, D. Mellström and A. Svanborg (G.S., University of Göteborg, Department of Obstetrics and Gynaecology, Sahlgrenska Sjukhuset, 413 45 Göteborg, Sweden)

Effects of oestriol on oscillation of circulating gonadotrophins during sleep in post-menopausal women.
H. Wauters, G. Buytaert and F. Uyttenbroeck (H.W., St. Camillus Kliniek, Lockaertstraat 10, Antwerpen, Belgium)

Effects of oestriol on lipid metabolism in climacteric women.
L. Rauramo (University of Turku, Department of Obstetrics and Gynaecology, Kaskenkatu II B, 20700 Turku 70, Finland)

Serum lipids and lipoproteins in 73-year-old women after treatment with oestriol.

G. Samsioe, N. Crona, D. Mellström and A. Svanborg (N.C., University of Göteborg, Department of Obstetrics and Gynaecology, Sahlgrenska Sjukhuset, 413 45 Göteborg, Sweden)

Endocrinological and clinical investigations in post-menopausal women following administration of vaginal cream containing oestriol.
A. A. Haspels, M. Luisi and P. M. Kicovic (A.A.H., Academisch Ziekenhuis Utrecht, Universiteitskliniek voor Obstetrie en Gynaecologie, Catharijnesingel 101, 3500 CG Utrecht, The Netherlands)

Use of oestriol cream in vaginal surgery in post-menopausal women.
J. Donnez and C. Lecart (J.D., Université Catholique de Louvain, Cliniques Universitaires Saint-Luc, Département de Gynécologie-Obstétrique, 10 avenue Hippocrate, 1200 Bruxelles, Belgium)

Treatment of post menopausal vaginal atrophy with Ovestin vaginal suppositories.
R. Trévoux and W. H. M. van der Velden (R.T., 31 rue de l'Assomption, 75016 Paris, France)

Free and conjugated oestriol plasma levels during vaginal oestriol treatment in post-menopausal women.
A. R. Genazzani, P. Inaudi, V. De Leo and S. La Marca (A.R.G., Università degli Studi di Siena, Cattedra di Patologia Ostetrica e Ginecologica, Via Pietro Mascagni 4, 53100 Siena, Italy)

V. Aspects of therapy – non-oestrogenic (Chairman: M. Neves-e-Castro)

Use of a sexual steroid (ORG OD 14) in the treatment of the climacteric syndrome.
P. R. Figueroa Casas (G.E.F.E.R., Casilla de Correo 999, 2000 Rosario (SF), Argentina)

Placebo-controlled cross-over study of effects of ORG OD 14 in climacteric women.
P. M. Kicovic, J. Cortes-Prieto, M. Luisi, S. Milojević and F. Franchi (P.M.K., Scoula di Specializzazione in Endocrinologia e Unità di Ricerce Endocrina del C.N.R. della Università degli Studi di Pisa, Pisa, Italy)

Double-blind cross-over study with ORG OD 14 in climacteric patients.
J. Nevinny-Stickel (Universitäts-Frauenklinik, Pulsstrasse 4-14, 1000 Berlin 19, West Germany)

The treatment of climacteric complaints with ORG OD 14, a new steroidal agent with no stimulatory effect on the endometrium.
R. Trévoux, P. Dieulangard and A. Blum (R. T., 31 rue de l'Assomption, 75016 Paris, France)

Study of the ovulation inhibiting properties of ORG OD 14.
P. Franchimont, F. Franchi, M. Luisi and P. M. Kicovic (P.M.K., Scoula di Specializzazione in Endocrinologia e Unità di Ricerca Endocrina del C.N.R. della Università degli Studi di Pisa, Pisa, Italy)

A short-term evaluation of sex hormone effect on skeletal metabolism by 24 hours whole body retention of diphosphonate.
D. M. Hart, I. Fogelman, R. G. Bessent, L. M. Smith and R. Lindsay (D.M.H., University of Glasgow, Division of Obstetrics and Gynaecology, Stobhill General Hospital, Glasgow G21 3UW, UK)

Medroxyprogesterone acetate in the treatment of the post-menopause syndrome.
J. Andor, E. Vögelin, H. Wyss, P. Schneider and K. Tscherne (J. A., Universitäts-Frauenklinik, Schanzenstrasse 46, 4000 Basel, Switzerland)

A double-blind cross-over study of the effect of norethisterone on climacteric symptoms.
M. E. L. Paterson (University of Leeds, Department of Obstetrics and Gynaecology, 17 Springfield Mount, Leeds LS2 9NG, UK)

The effect of a new oral progestogen, ORG 2969, on circulating FSH, LH and prolactin in peri-menopausal patients.
P. Franchimont and P. M. Kicovic (P.M.K., Scoula di Specializzazione in Endocrinologia e Unità di Picerca Endocrina del C.N.R. della Università degli Studi di Pisa, Pisa, Italy)

Evaluation of a continuous oestrogen–progestogen regimen for climacteric complaints: clinical, morphological and hormonal aspects.
L.-Å. Mattsson, G. Cullberg and G. Samsioe (L.-Å.M., Östra Sjukhuset, Department of Obstetrics and Gynaecology, 416 85 Göteborg, Sweden)

Psychological changes effected by oestrogen–progestogen and clonidine treatment in climacteric women.

L. C. Gerdes, E. W. W. Sonnendecker and E. S. Polakow (E. W. W. S., University of the Witwatersrand, Medical School, Department of Obstetrics and Gynaecology, Johannesburg Hospital, Jubilee Road, Parktown 2193, South Africa)

Ethamsylate, a non-hormonal alternative for the treatment of climacteric flushing.

R. F. Harrison (University of Dublin, Trinity College, Department of Obstetrics and Gynaecology, Rotunda Hospital, Dublin, Ireland)

Clinical and biological study of veralipride treatment of climacteric hot flushes.

S. Wesel, M. L'Hermite-Baleriaux and M. L'Hermite (S. W., Hôpital de Braine-l'Alleud-Waterloo, 35 rue Wayez, 1420 Braine-l'Alleud, Belgium)

Management of pre-menopausal uterine pathology with lynestrenol.

C. Babuna (Istanbul University, Faculty of Medicine, Department of Obstetrics and Gynecology, Istanbul, Turkey)

POSTERS

Influence of dehydroepiandrosterone administration on serum hormones in post-menopausal women.

K. Araki, Y. Tomita, K. Akasofu and E. Nishida (K. A., Kanazawa University School of Medicine, Department of Obstetrics and Gynaecology, 13-1 Takara-machi, Kanazawa 920, Japan)

Oestrogen profiles after surgical menopause; effects of the early administration of oestrogen.

D. H. Barlow, H. P. McEwan, R. Fleming and J. R. T. Coutts (D. H. B., University of Glasgow, University Department of Obstetrics and Gynaecology, Royal Maternity Hospital, Rottenrow, Glasgow G4 0NA, UK)

Favourable effect of natural oestrogens on the menopausal epithelium.

G. Gimes and R. Gimes (G. G., 1082 Ülloi u. 78, II. Department of Obstetrics and Gynaecology, Budapest, Hungary)

Therapeutic effect of cyproterone acetate on climacteric complaints.
R. Gimes and S. Csömör (R. G., 1088 Baross u. 27, I. Department of Obstetrics and Gynaecology, Budapest, Hungary)

Oestrone and oestradiol plasma levels after the administration of conjugated oestrogens by different routes.
V. M. Jasonni, L. la Marca, G. Lesi, A. P. Ferraretti, O. Magrini, A. Guidi, G. Cassani, C. Bulletti and C. Flamigni (V.M.J., Università di Bologna, Fisiopatologia della Riproduzione, Clinica Ostetrica e Ginecologica, Massarenti 13, 40138 Bologna, Italy)

The Center for Climacteric Studies.
M. Notelovitz, K. Putney, L. McKenzie and R. Tesar (M. N., The Center for Climacteric Studies, University of Florida, The Professional Center, 901 NW 8th Avenue, Suite B-1, Gainesville, FL 32601, USA)

The menstrual cycle: age-related changes in older women.
L. Sexton, E. A. Lenton and I. D. Cooke (L.S., University of Sheffield, Department of Obstetrics and Gynaecology, Jessop Hospital for Women, Sheffield S3 7RE, UK)

Basal and LRH and LRH-analogue stimulated plasma glycoprotein hormone A-subunit in five post-menopausal women.
M. L. Batrinos, S. Pitoulis, M. Anapliotou and C. Panitsa-Faflia (M.L.B., University of Athens, Department of Pharmacology, Athens Goudi 609, Greece)

Survey of sampling methods for endometrial cytology with special reference to the Isaacs cell sampler.
O.-E. Iversen and E. Segadal (O.-E.I., University of Bergen, Department of Obstetrics and Gynaecology, Haukeland Hospital, Bergen, Norway)

Hormonal pattern in men from puberty to old age.
G. Sorcini, G. Matarazzo, E. Fabietti, F. Abbadessa, C. Felicetti, M. Genderini, S. Marini and A. Rovigatti (G.S., Università di Roma, Istituto di Clinica Medica Generale e Terapia Medica V, Policlinico Umberto, 1, 00100 Roma, Italy)

Index